Accident

Record Book ©

Personal

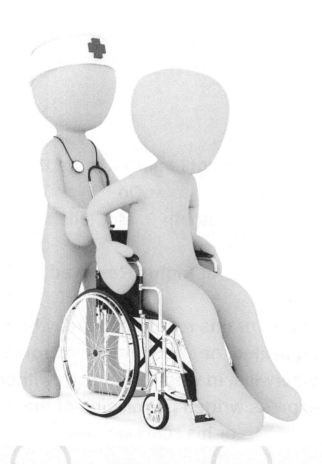

Kenneth R. McClelland

Accident / Injury Record Book
~oOo~
Kenneth R. McClelland

~ Accident / Injury Record Book ~

This accident / injury, record book, belongs to, and is the personal private property of: _____

_____

If found or left unattended, please contact the owner of this record book, at: _____

_____

Date of accident or injury:_____ **Time:**_____

Where did your injury occur:_____

_____

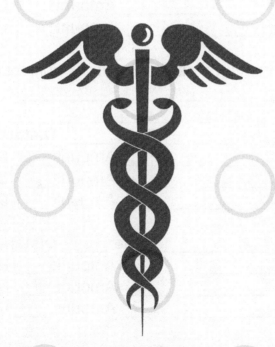

NOTE: *Continue to update this pain tracking record book so that a more detailed timeline of your ailment's progression or regression may be established.*

~ Accident / Injury Record Book ~

Primary Hospital or Medical Facility, location & contact information: _____
_____
_____

Appt. Date:_____ **Time**:_____ **Distance**: _____
Prescription:_____ Amount:____ Dose:_____
Prescription:_____ Amount:____ Dose:_____
Prescription: _____ Amount:____ Dose:_____
Prescription: _____ Amount:____ Dose:_____

Hospital or Medical Facility, location & contact info: _____
_____
_____

Appt. Date:_____ **Time**:_____ **Distance**: _____
Prescription:_____ Amount:____ Dose:_____
Prescription:_____ Amount:____ Dose:_____
Prescription: _____ Amount:____ Dose:_____

Primary Physician's name, location & contact info: _____
_____
_____

Appt. Date:_____ **Time**:_____ **Distance**: _____
Prescription: _____ Amount:____ Dose:_____
Prescription: _____ Amount:____ Dose:_____
Prescription: _____ Amount:____ Dose:_____

Appt. Date:_____ **Time**:_____ **Distance**: _____
Prescription: _____ Amount:____ Dose:_____
Prescription: _____ Amount:____ Dose:_____
Prescription: _____ Amount:____ Dose:_____

Appt. Date:_____ **Time**:_____ **Distance**: _____
Prescription: _____ Amount:____ Dose:_____
Prescription: _____ Amount:____ Dose:_____
Prescription: _____ Amount:____ Dose:_____

4

~ Accident / Injury Record Book ~

Primary Physician's name, location & contact info (cont.):
_____
_____

Appt. Date:_____ **Time**:_____ **Distance**:_____
Prescription: _____ Amount:____ Dose:_____
Prescription: _____ Amount:____ Dose:_____
Prescription: _____ Amount:____ Dose:_____

Appt. Date:_____ **Time**:_____ **Distance**:_____
Prescription: _____ Amount:____ Dose:_____
Prescription: _____ Amount:____ Dose:_____
Prescription: _____ Amount:____ Dose:_____

Appt. Date:_____ **Time**:_____ **Distance**:_____
Prescription: _____ Amount:____ Dose:_____
Prescription: _____ Amount:____ Dose:_____
Prescription: _____ Amount:____ Dose:_____

Appt. Date:_____ **Time**:_____ **Distance**:_____
Prescription: _____ Amount:____ Dose:_____
Prescription: _____ Amount:____ Dose:_____

Specialist's name, specialty & contact info:_____
_____
_____

Appt. Date:_____ **Time**:_____ **Distance:**_____
Prescription: _____ Amount:____ Dose:_____
Prescription: _____ Amount:____ Dose:_____

Appt. Date:_____ **Time**:_____ **Distance**:_____
Prescription: _____ Amount:____ Dose:_____
Prescription: _____ Amount:____ Dose:_____

Appt. Date:_____ **Time**:_____ **Distance**:_____
Prescription: _____ Amount:____ Dose:_____

~ Accident / Injury Record Book ~

Specialist's name, specialty & contact info:_____
_____
_____

Appt. Date:_____ **Time**:_____ **Distance**:_____
Prescription:_____ Amount:____ Dose:_____
Prescription:_____ Amount:____ Dose:_____

Appt. Date:_____ **Time**:_____ **Distance**:_____
Prescription:_____ Amount:____ Dose:_____

Appt. Date:_____ **Time**:_____ **Distance**:_____
Prescription:_____ Amount:____ Dose:_____

Specialist's name, specialty & contact info:_____
_____
_____

Appt. Date:_____ **Time**:_____ **Distance**:_____
Prescription:_____ Amount:____ Dose:_____
Prescription:_____ Amount:____ Dose:_____

Appt. Date:_____ **Time**:_____ **Distance**:_____
Prescription:_____ Amount:____ Dose:_____

Appt. Date:_____ **Time**:_____ **Distance**:_____
Prescription:_____ Amount:____ Dose:_____

Specialist's name, specialty & contact info:_____
_____
_____

Appt. Date:_____ **Time**:_____ **Distance**:_____
Prescription:_____ Amount:____ Dose:_____
Prescription:_____ Amount:____ Dose:_____

Appt. Date:_____ **Time**:_____ **Distance**:_____
Prescription:_____ Amount:____ Dose:_____

~ Accident / Injury Record Book ~

Physical Therapist name & contact info:_____

_____

Appt. Date:_____ **Time**:_____ **Distance**:_____
Appt. Date:_____ Appt. Date:_____
Appt. Date:_____ Appt. Date:_____
Appt. Date:_____ Appt. Date:_____

Physical Therapist name & contact info:_____

_____

Appt. Date:_____ **Time**:_____ **Distance**:_____
Appt. Date:_____ Appt. Date:_____
Appt. Date:_____ Appt. Date:_____
Appt. Date:_____ Appt. Date:_____

Physical Therapist name & contact info:_____

_____

Appt. Date:_____ **Time**:_____ **Distance**:_____
Appt. Date:_____ Appt. Date:_____
Appt. Date:_____ Appt. Date:_____
Appt. Date:_____ Appt. Date:_____

MRI / X-ray Ctr. name & contact info: _____

_____

Appt. Date:_____ **Time**:_____ **Distance**:_____
Appt. Date:_____ Appt. Date: _____
Appt. Date:_____ Appt. Date: _____

MRI / X-ray Ctr. name & contact info:_____

_____

Appt. Date:_____ **Time**:_____ **Distance**:_____
Appt. Date:_____ Appt. Date: _____

MRI / X-ray Ctr. name & contact info: _____

_____

Appt. Date:_____ **Time**:_____ **Distance**:_____

~ Accident / Injury Record Book ~

Lab Work / Diagnostic Ctr. name & contact info:_____

_____

Appt. Date:_____ **Time**:_____ **Distance**: _____
Appt. Date:_____ Appt. Date:_____
Appt. Date:_____ Appt. Date:_____

Lab Work / Diagnostic Ctr. name & contact info:_____

_____

Appt. Date:_____ **Time**:_____ **Distance**: _____
Appt. Date:_____ Appt. Date:_____
Appt. Date:_____ Appt. Date:_____

Lab Work / Diagnostic Ctr. name & contact info:_____

_____

Appt. Date:_____ **Time**:_____ **Distance**: _____
Appt. Date:_____ Appt. Date:_____
Appt. Date:_____ Appt. Date:_____

Pharmacy name & contact info:_____

_____

Pharmacy name & contact info:_____

_____

_____

Misc. info:_____

Misc. info:_____

Misc. info._____

_____

_____

_____

_____

~ Accident / Injury Record Book ~

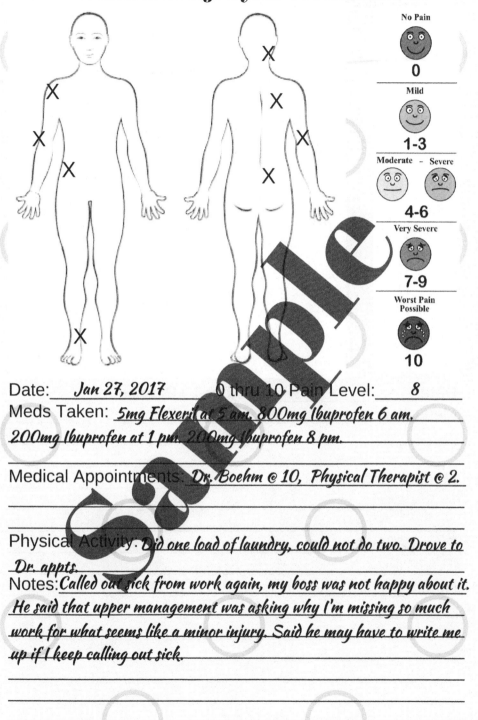

No Pain
0

Mild
1-3

Moderate – Severe
4-6

Very Severe
7-9

Worst Pain Possible
10

Date: *Jan 27, 2017*   0 thru 10 Pain Level: _____8_____

Meds Taken: *5mg Flexeril at 5 am, 800mg Ibuprofen 6 am, 200mg Ibuprofen at 1 pm, 200mg Ibuprofen 8 pm.*

Medical Appointments: *Dr. Boehm @ 10, Physical Therapist @ 2.*

Physical Activity: *Did one load of laundry, could not do two. Drove to Dr. appts.*

Notes: *Called out sick from work again, my boss was not happy about it. He said that upper management was asking why I'm missing so much work for what seems like a minor injury. Said he may have to write me up if I keep calling out sick.*

Additional notes on page: # _____

~ Accident / Injury Record Book ~

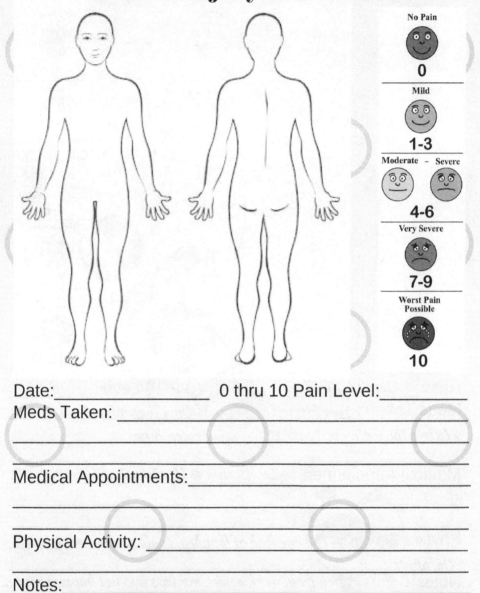

No Pain
0

Mild
1-3

Moderate – Severe
4-6

Very Severe
7-9

Worst Pain Possible
10

Date:_____ 0 thru 10 Pain Level:_____

Meds Taken: _____

_____

Medical Appointments:_____

_____

_____

Physical Activity: _____

_____

Notes:_____

_____

_____

_____

_____

_____

_____

Additional notes on page: # _____

~ Accident / Injury Record Book ~

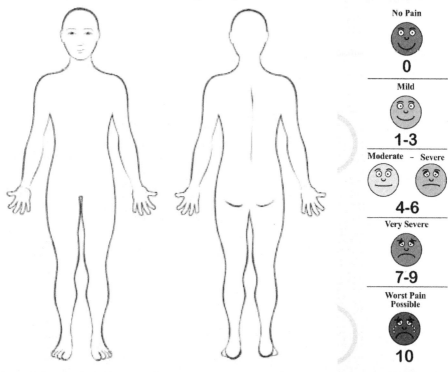

No Pain
0

Mild
1-3

Moderate – Severe
4-6

Very Severe
7-9

Worst Pain Possible
10

Date:_____ 0 thru 10 Pain Level:_____

Meds Taken: _____

_____

_____

Medical Appointments:_____

_____

_____

Physical Activity: _____

_____

Notes:_____

_____

_____

_____

_____

_____

_____

Additional notes on page: # _____

~ Accident / Injury Record Book ~

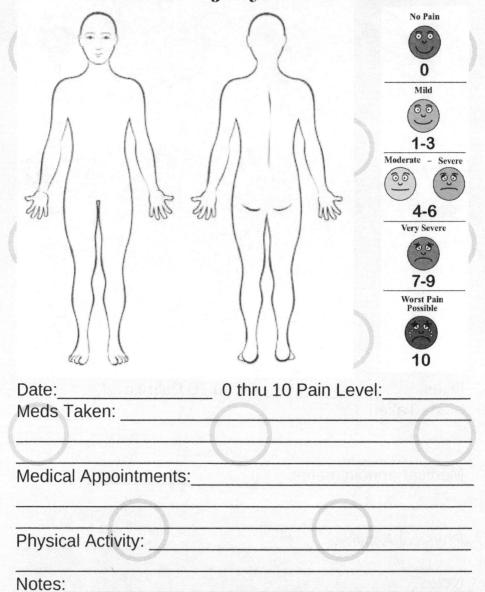

No Pain
0

Mild
1-3

Moderate – Severe
4-6

Very Severe
7-9

Worst Pain Possible
10

Date:_____ 0 thru 10 Pain Level:_____

Meds Taken: _____
_____
_____

Medical Appointments:_____
_____
_____

Physical Activity: _____
_____

Notes:_____
_____
_____
_____
_____
_____
_____

Additional notes on page: # _____

~ Accident / Injury Record Book ~

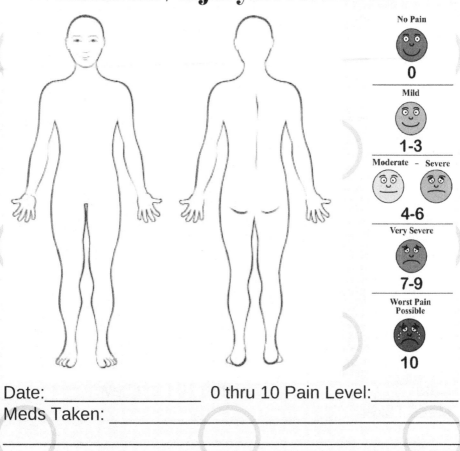

No Pain

0

Mild

1-3

Moderate – Severe

4-6

Very Severe

7-9

Worst Pain Possible

10

Date:_____ 0 thru 10 Pain Level:_____

Meds Taken: _____
_____

Medical Appointments:_____
_____

Physical Activity: _____

Notes:_____
_____
_____
_____
_____
_____

Additional notes on page: # _____

~ Accident / Injury Record Book ~

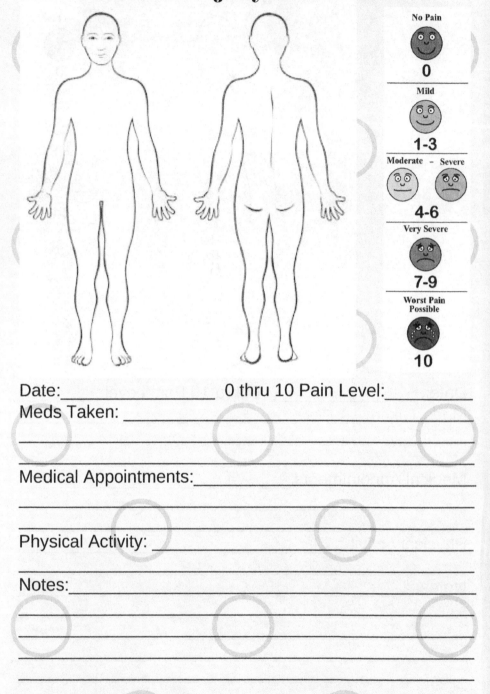

No Pain
0

Mild
1-3

Moderate – Severe
4-6

Very Severe
7-9

Worst Pain Possible
10

Date:_____ 0 thru 10 Pain Level:_____

Meds Taken: _____

_____

Medical Appointments:_____

_____

Physical Activity: _____

_____

Notes:_____

_____

_____

_____

_____

_____

Additional notes on page: # _____

~ Accident / Injury Record Book ~

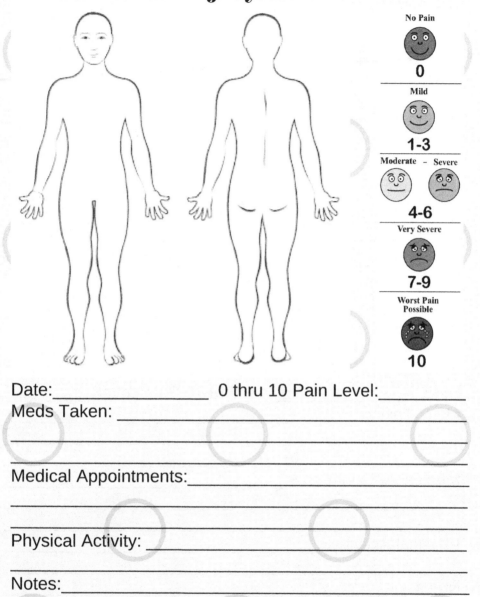

No Pain
0

Mild
1-3

Moderate – Severe
4-6

Very Severe
7-9

Worst Pain Possible
10

Date:_____ 0 thru 10 Pain Level:_____

Meds Taken: _____
_____
_____

Medical Appointments:_____
_____
_____

Physical Activity: _____
_____

Notes:_____
_____
_____
_____
_____
_____
_____

Additional notes on page: # _____

~ Accident / Injury Record Book ~

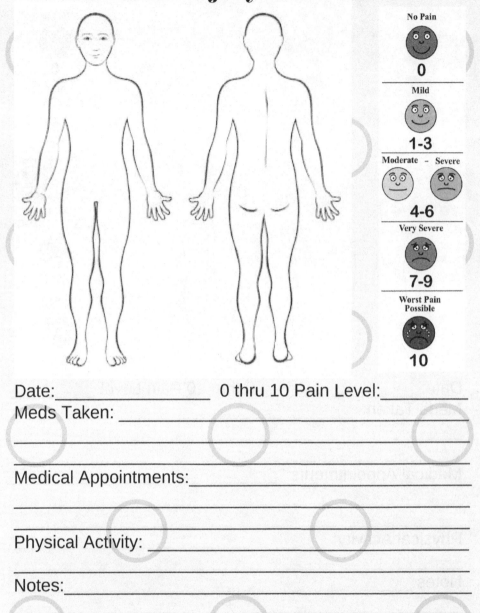

No Pain
0

Mild
1-3

Moderate – Severe
4-6

Very Severe
7-9

Worst Pain Possible
10

Date:_____ 0 thru 10 Pain Level:_____

Meds Taken: _____

_____

Medical Appointments:_____

_____

Physical Activity: _____

_____

Notes:_____

_____

_____

_____

_____

_____

Additional notes on page: # _____

~ Accident / Injury Record Book ~

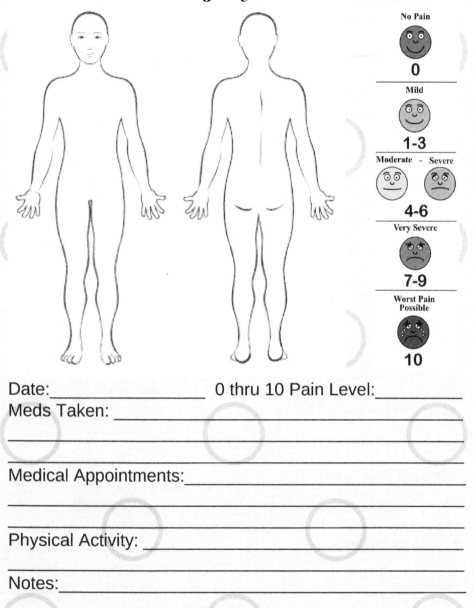

No Pain
0

Mild
1-3

Moderate – Severe
4-6

Very Severe
7-9

Worst Pain Possible
10

Date:_____ 0 thru 10 Pain Level:_____

Meds Taken: _____
_____

Medical Appointments:_____
_____

Physical Activity: _____

Notes:_____
_____
_____
_____
_____
_____

Additional notes on page: # _____

~ Accident / Injury Record Book ~

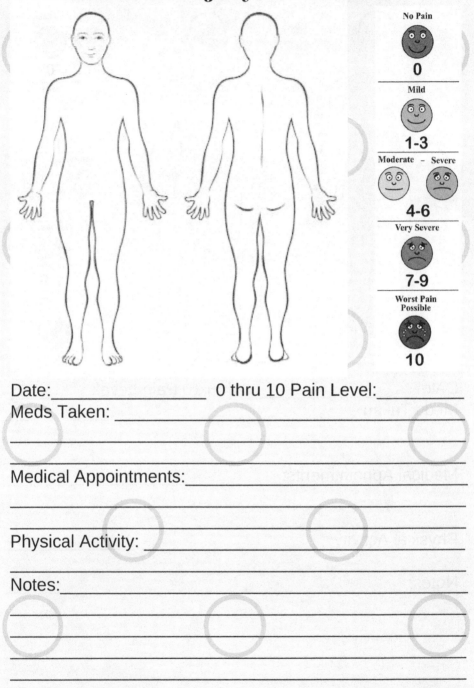

No Pain
0

Mild
1-3

Moderate – Severe
4-6

Very Severe
7-9

Worst Pain Possible
10

Date:_____ 0 thru 10 Pain Level:_____

Meds Taken: _____
_____

Medical Appointments:_____
_____
_____

Physical Activity: _____
_____

Notes:_____
_____
_____
_____
_____
_____
_____

Additional notes on page: # _____

~ Accident / Injury Record Book ~

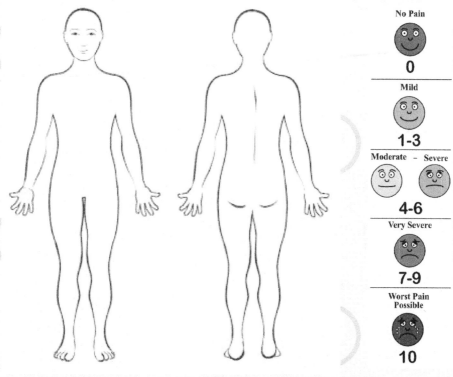

No Pain
0

Mild
1-3

Moderate – Severe
4-6

Very Severe
7-9

Worst Pain Possible
10

Date:_____ 0 thru 10 Pain Level:_____

Meds Taken: _____

_____

_____

Medical Appointments:_____

_____

Physical Activity: _____

_____

Notes:_____

_____

_____

_____

_____

_____

_____

_____

Additional notes on page: # _____

~ Accident / Injury Record Book ~

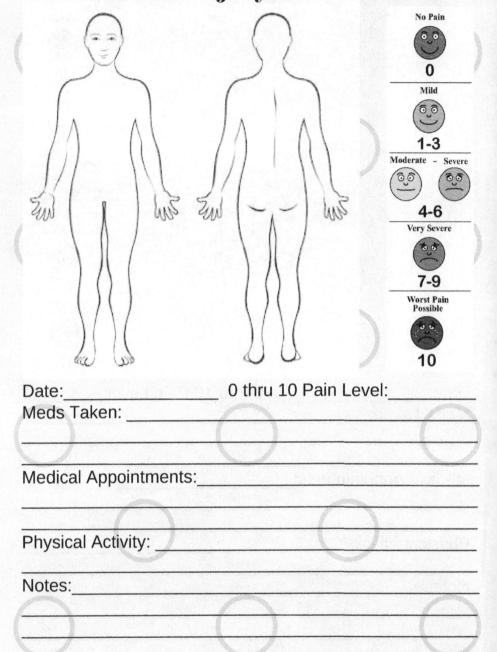

No Pain
0

Mild
1-3

Moderate – Severe
4-6

Very Severe
7-9

Worst Pain Possible
10

Date:_____ 0 thru 10 Pain Level:_____

Meds Taken: _____
_____
_____

Medical Appointments:_____
_____
_____

Physical Activity: _____
_____

Notes:_____
_____
_____
_____
_____
_____
_____

Additional notes on page: # _____

~ Accident / Injury Record Book ~

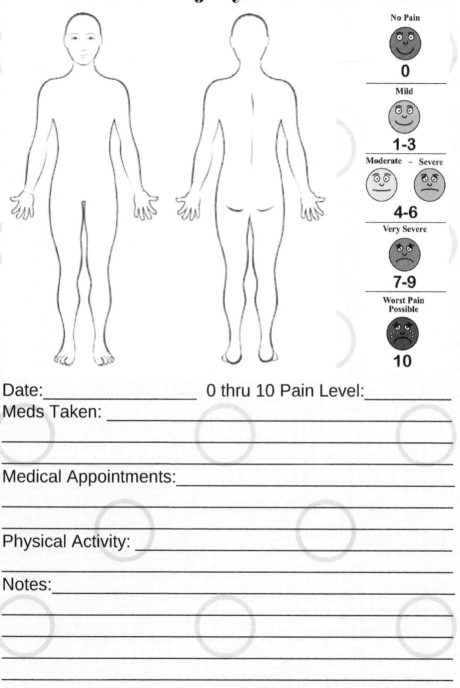

No Pain

0

Mild

1-3

Moderate – Severe

4-6

Very Severe

7-9

Worst Pain Possible

10

Date:_____ 0 thru 10 Pain Level:_____

Meds Taken: _____

_____

_____

Medical Appointments:_____

_____

_____

Physical Activity: _____

_____

Notes:_____

_____

_____

_____

_____

_____

_____

Additional notes on page: # _____

~ Accident / Injury Record Book ~

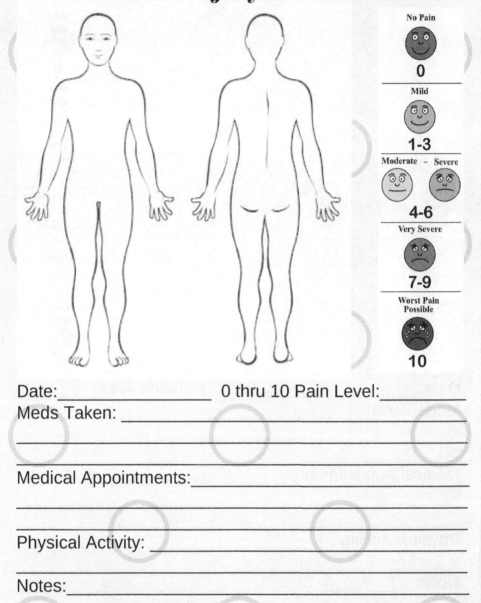

Date:_____ 0 thru 10 Pain Level:_____

Meds Taken: _____
_____
_____

Medical Appointments:_____
_____
_____

Physical Activity: _____
_____

Notes:_____
_____
_____
_____
_____
_____
_____

Additional notes on page: # _____

~ Accident / Injury Record Book ~

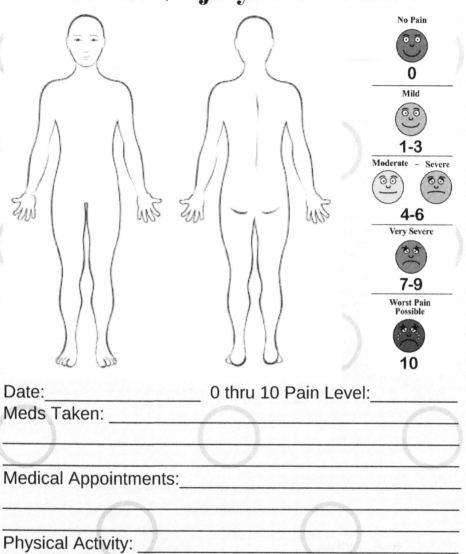

No Pain
0

Mild
1-3

Moderate – Severe
4-6

Very Severe
7-9

Worst Pain Possible
10

Date:_____ 0 thru 10 Pain Level:_____

Meds Taken: _____
_____
_____

Medical Appointments:_____
_____
_____

Physical Activity: _____
_____

Notes:_____
_____
_____
_____
_____
_____
_____

Additional notes on page: # _____

~ Accident / Injury Record Book ~

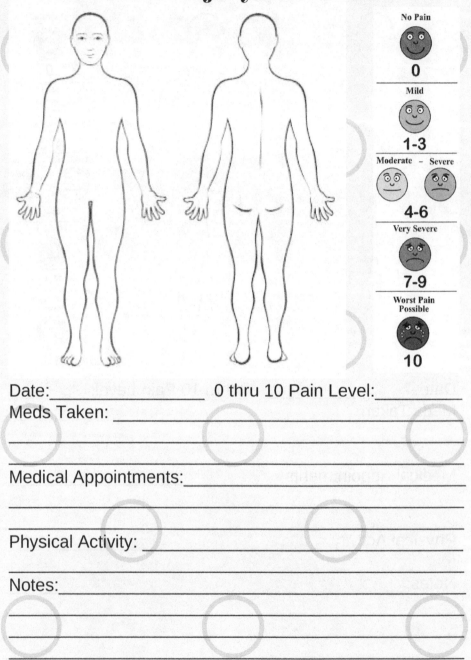

No Pain
0

Mild
1-3

Moderate – Severe
4-6

Very Severe
7-9

Worst Pain Possible
10

Date:_____ 0 thru 10 Pain Level:_____

Meds Taken: _____

_____

Medical Appointments:_____

_____

Physical Activity: _____

_____

Notes:_____

_____

_____

_____

_____

_____

_____

Additional notes on page: # _____

~ Accident / Injury Record Book ~

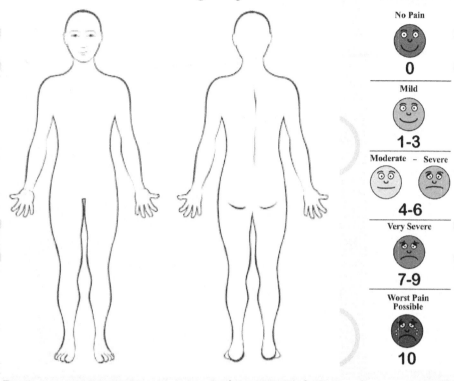

No Pain
0

Mild
1-3

Moderate – Severe
4-6

Very Severe
7-9

Worst Pain Possible
10

Date:_____ 0 thru 10 Pain Level:_____

Meds Taken: _____
_____

Medical Appointments:_____
_____

Physical Activity: _____
_____

Notes:_____
_____
_____
_____
_____
_____
_____

Additional notes on page: # _____

~ Accident / Injury Record Book ~

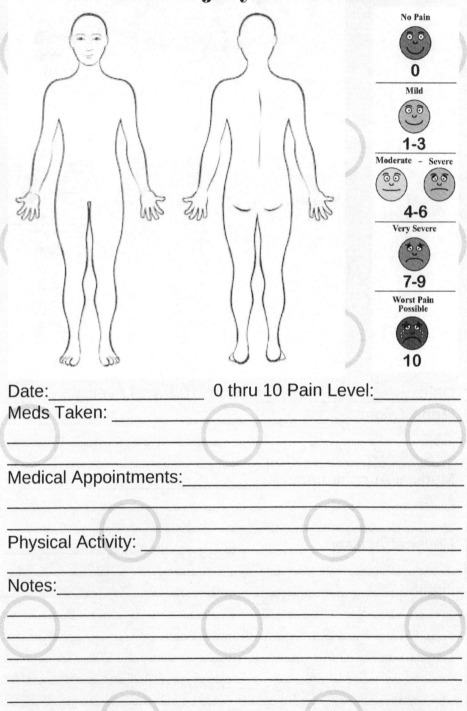

No Pain
0

Mild
1-3

Moderate – Severe
4-6

Very Severe
7-9

Worst Pain Possible
10

Date:_____ 0 thru 10 Pain Level:_____

Meds Taken: _____
_____

Medical Appointments:_____
_____
_____

Physical Activity: _____
_____

Notes:_____
_____
_____
_____
_____
_____
_____

Additional notes on page: # _____

~ Accident / Injury Record Book ~

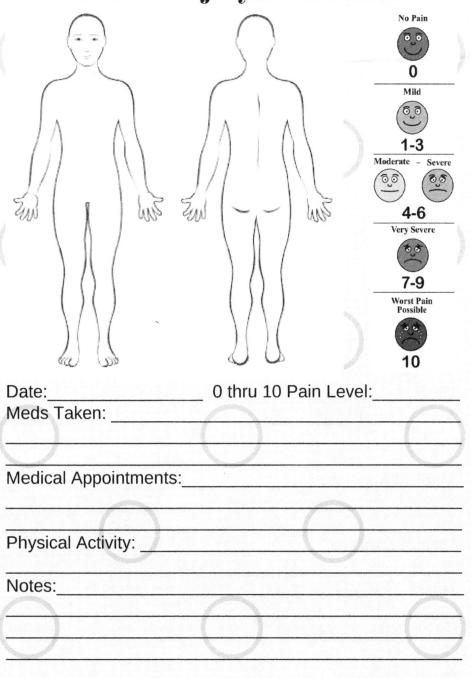

No Pain
0

Mild
1-3

Moderate – Severe
4-6

Very Severe
7-9

Worst Pain Possible
10

Date:_____ 0 thru 10 Pain Level:_____

Meds Taken: _____
_____
_____

Medical Appointments:_____
_____
_____

Physical Activity: _____
_____

Notes:_____
_____
_____
_____
_____
_____
_____

Additional notes on page: # _____

~ Accident / Injury Record Book ~

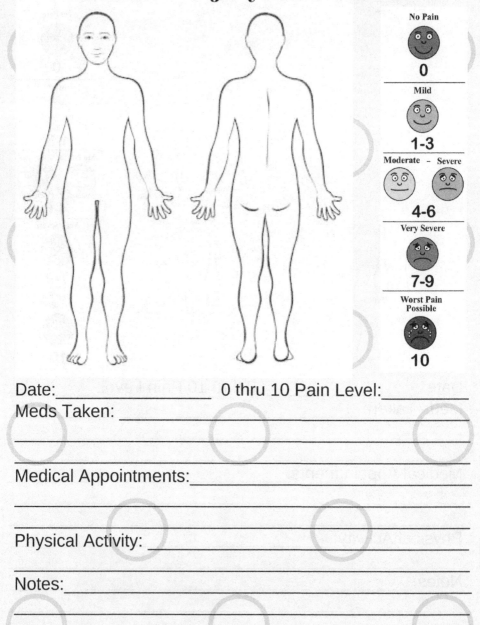

No Pain
0

Mild
1-3

Moderate – Severe
4-6

Very Severe
7-9

Worst Pain Possible
10

Date:_____ 0 thru 10 Pain Level:_____

Meds Taken: _____
_____

Medical Appointments:_____
_____

Physical Activity: _____
_____

Notes:_____
_____
_____
_____
_____
_____
_____
_____

Additional notes on page: # _____

~ Accident / Injury Record Book ~

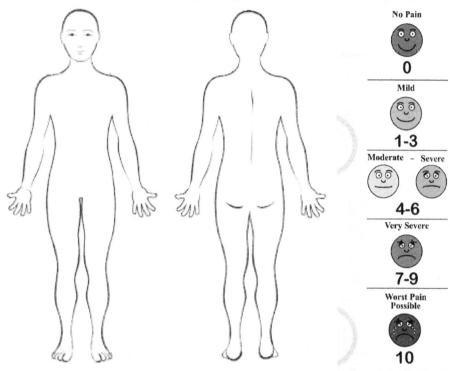

No Pain
0

Mild
1-3

Moderate – Severe
4-6

Very Severe
7-9

Worst Pain Possible
10

Date:_____ 0 thru 10 Pain Level:_____

Meds Taken: _____
_____
_____

Medical Appointments:_____
_____
_____

Physical Activity: _____
_____

Notes:_____
_____
_____
_____
_____
_____
_____
_____

Additional notes on page: # _____

~ Accident / Injury Record Book ~

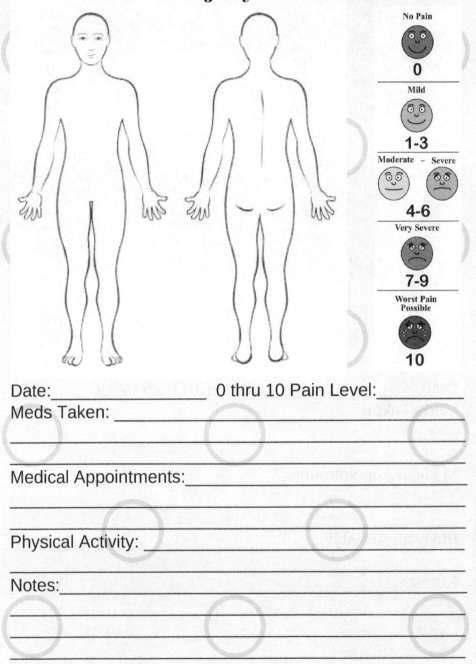

No Pain
0

Mild
1-3

Moderate – Severe
4-6

Very Severe
7-9

Worst Pain Possible
10

Date:_____ 0 thru 10 Pain Level:_____

Meds Taken: _____
_____

Medical Appointments:_____
_____
_____

Physical Activity: _____
_____

Notes:_____
_____
_____
_____
_____
_____
_____

Additional notes on page: # _____

~ Accident / Injury Record Book ~

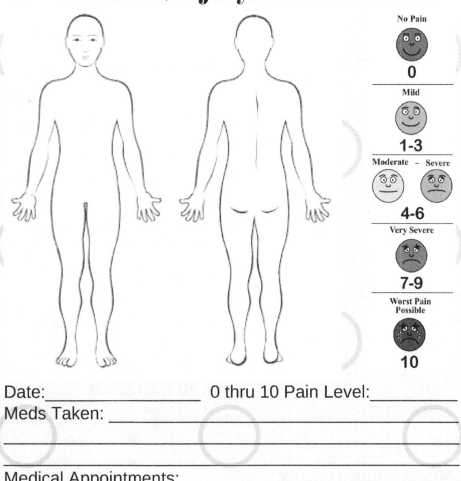

No Pain
0

Mild
1-3

Moderate – Severe
4-6

Very Severe
7-9

Worst Pain Possible
10

Date:_____ 0 thru 10 Pain Level:_____

Meds Taken: _____
_____

Medical Appointments:_____
_____

Physical Activity: _____
_____

Notes:_____
_____
_____
_____
_____
_____
_____

Additional notes on page: # _____

~ Accident / Injury Record Book ~

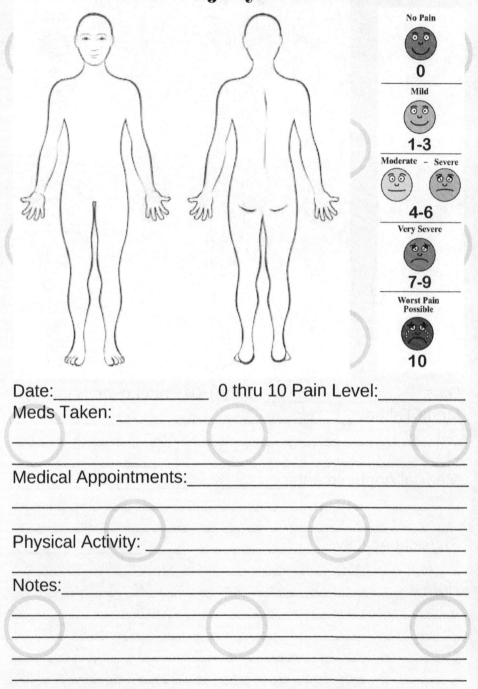

No Pain

0

Mild

1-3

Moderate – Severe

4-6

Very Severe

7-9

Worst Pain Possible

10

Date:_____ 0 thru 10 Pain Level:_____

Meds Taken: _____

_____

_____

Medical Appointments:_____

_____

_____

Physical Activity: _____

_____

Notes:_____

_____

_____

_____

_____

_____

_____

Additional notes on page: # _____

~ Accident / Injury Record Book ~

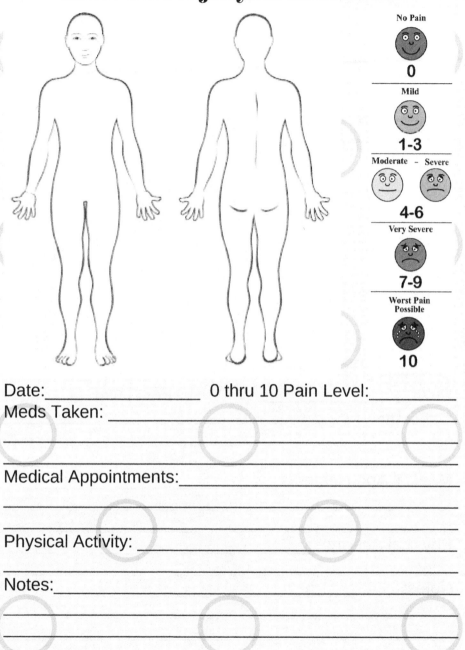

No Pain
0

Mild
1-3

Moderate – Severe
4-6

Very Severe
7-9

Worst Pain Possible
10

Date:_____ 0 thru 10 Pain Level:_____

Meds Taken: _____
_____
_____

Medical Appointments:_____
_____
_____

Physical Activity: _____
_____

Notes:_____
_____
_____
_____
_____
_____
_____
_____

Additional notes on page: # _____

~ Accident / Injury Record Book ~

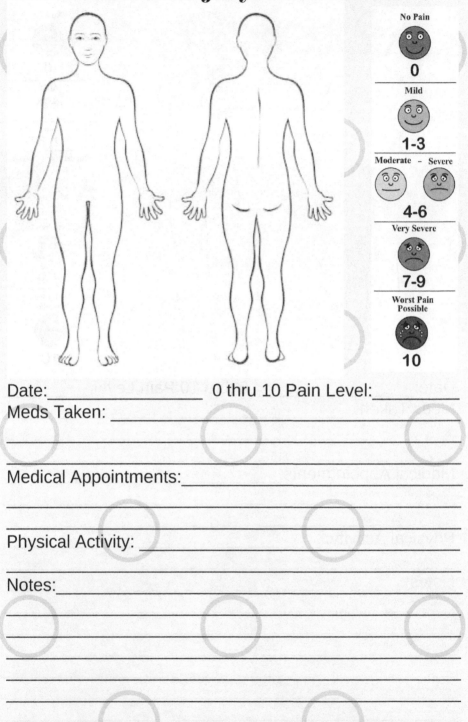

No Pain
0

Mild
1-3

Moderate – Severe
4-6

Very Severe
7-9

Worst Pain Possible
10

Date:_____ 0 thru 10 Pain Level:_____

Meds Taken: _____

_____

Medical Appointments:_____

_____

Physical Activity: _____

_____

Notes:_____

_____

_____

_____

_____

_____

_____

Additional notes on page: # _____

~ Accident / Injury Record Book ~

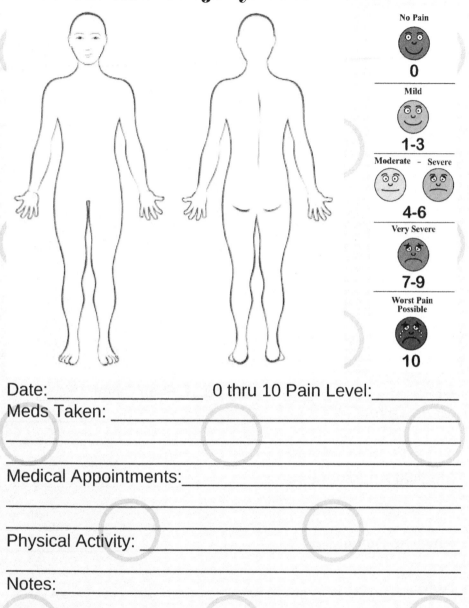

No Pain
0

Mild
1-3

Moderate – Severe
4-6

Very Severe
7-9

Worst Pain Possible
10

Date:_____ 0 thru 10 Pain Level:_____

Meds Taken: _____
_____
_____

Medical Appointments:_____
_____
_____

Physical Activity: _____
_____

Notes:_____
_____
_____
_____
_____
_____
_____

Additional notes on page: # _____

~ Accident / Injury Record Book ~

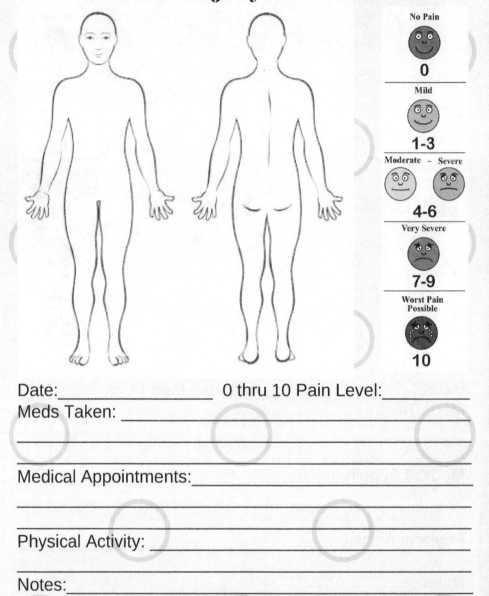

No Pain

0

Mild

1-3

Moderate – Severe

4-6

Very Severe

7-9

Worst Pain Possible

10

Date:_____ 0 thru 10 Pain Level:_____

Meds Taken: _____

_____

Medical Appointments:_____

_____

Physical Activity: _____

_____

Notes:_____

_____

_____

_____

_____

_____

_____

Additional notes on page: # _____

~ Accident / Injury Record Book ~

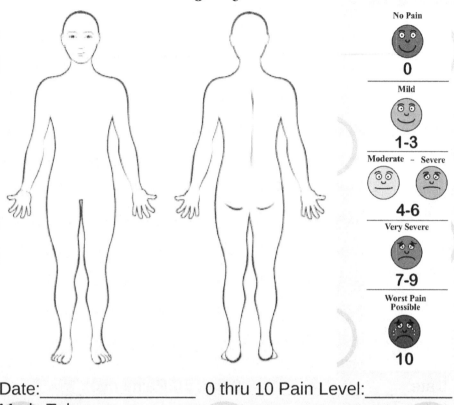

No Pain

0

Mild

1-3

Moderate – Severe

4-6

Very Severe

7-9

Worst Pain Possible

10

Date:_____ 0 thru 10 Pain Level:_____

Meds Taken: _____

_____

Medical Appointments:_____

_____

Physical Activity: _____

_____

Notes:_____

_____

_____

_____

_____

_____

Additional notes on page: # _____

~ Accident / Injury Record Book ~

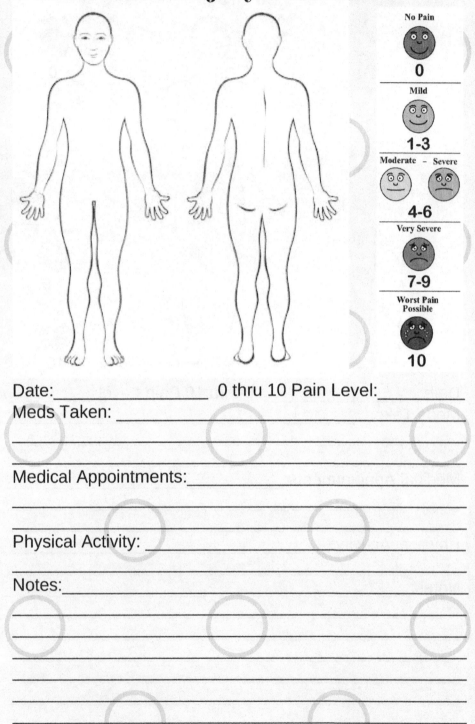

No Pain

0

Mild

1-3

Moderate – Severe

4-6

Very Severe

7-9

Worst Pain Possible

10

Date:_____ 0 thru 10 Pain Level:_____

Meds Taken: _____
_____

Medical Appointments:_____
_____
_____

Physical Activity: _____
_____

Notes:_____
_____
_____
_____
_____
_____
_____

Additional notes on page: # _____

~ Accident / Injury Record Book ~

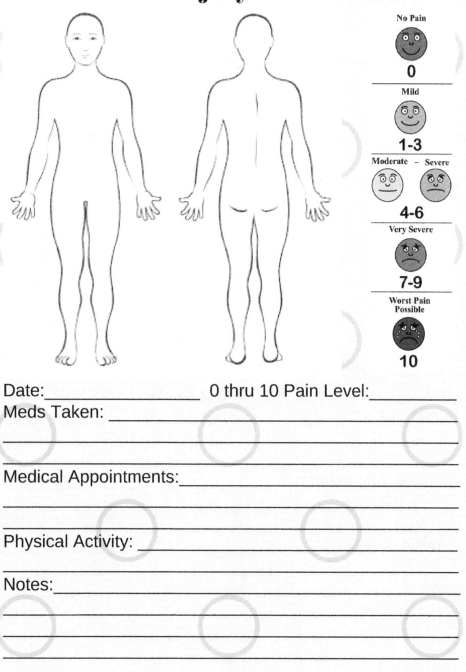

No Pain
0

Mild
1-3

Moderate – Severe
4-6

Very Severe
7-9

Worst Pain Possible
10

Date:_____ 0 thru 10 Pain Level:_____

Meds Taken: _____
_____
_____

Medical Appointments:_____
_____
_____

Physical Activity: _____
_____

Notes:_____
_____
_____
_____
_____
_____
_____

Additional notes on page: # _____

~ Accident / Injury Record Book ~

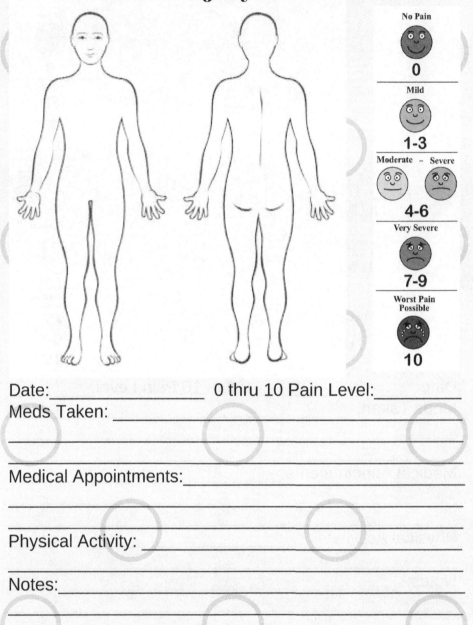

No Pain

0

Mild

1-3

Moderate – Severe

4-6

Very Severe

7-9

Worst Pain Possible

10

Date:_____ 0 thru 10 Pain Level:_____

Meds Taken: _____

_____

Medical Appointments:_____

_____

_____

Physical Activity: _____

_____

Notes:_____

_____

_____

_____

_____

_____

_____

_____

Additional notes on page: # _____

~ Accident / Injury Record Book ~

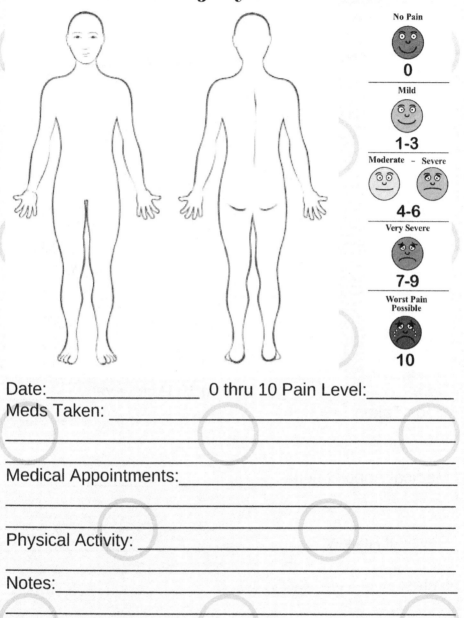

No Pain
0

Mild
1-3

Moderate – Severe
4-6

Very Severe
7-9

Worst Pain Possible
10

Date:_____ 0 thru 10 Pain Level:_____

Meds Taken: _____
_____

Medical Appointments:_____
_____
_____

Physical Activity: _____
_____

Notes:_____
_____
_____
_____
_____
_____
_____

Additional notes on page: # _____

~ Accident / Injury Record Book ~

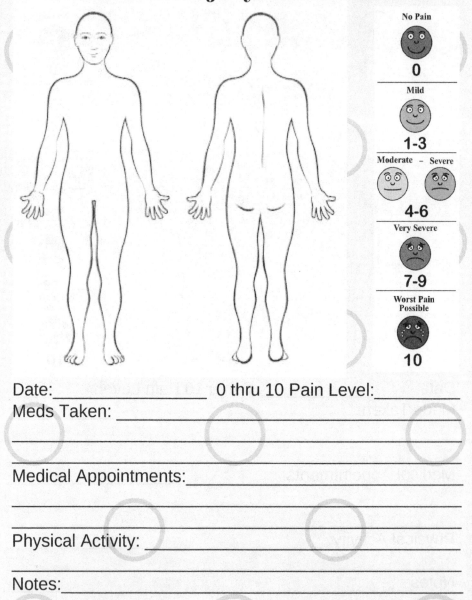

No Pain
0

Mild
1-3

Moderate – Severe
4-6

Very Severe
7-9

Worst Pain Possible
10

Date:_____ 0 thru 10 Pain Level:_____

Meds Taken: _____
_____
_____

Medical Appointments:_____
_____
_____

Physical Activity: _____
_____

Notes:_____
_____
_____
_____
_____
_____
_____
_____

Additional notes on page: # _____

~ Accident / Injury Record Book ~

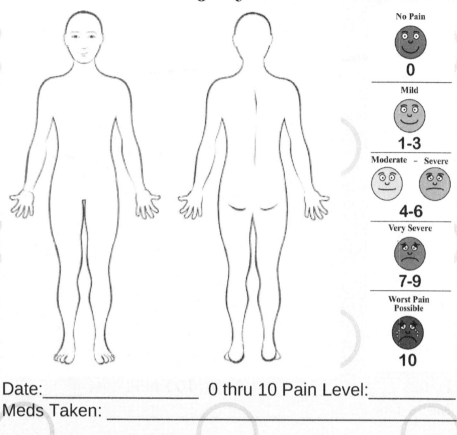

No Pain
0

Mild
1-3

Moderate ~ Severe
4-6

Very Severe
7-9

Worst Pain Possible
10

Date:_____ 0 thru 10 Pain Level:_____

Meds Taken: _____
_____

Medical Appointments:_____
_____

Physical Activity: _____
_____

Notes:_____
_____
_____
_____
_____
_____
_____
_____

Additional notes on page: # _____

~ Accident / Injury Record Book ~

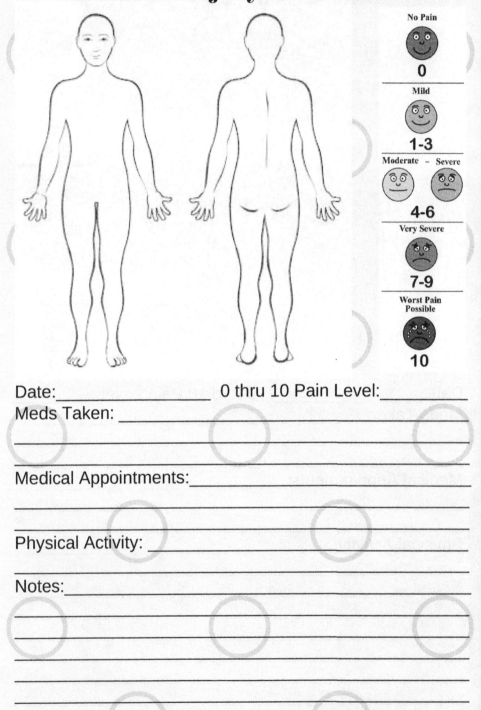

No Pain
0

Mild
1-3

Moderate – Severe
4-6

Very Severe
7-9

Worst Pain Possible
10

Date:_____ 0 thru 10 Pain Level:_____

Meds Taken: _____
_____

Medical Appointments:_____
_____
_____

Physical Activity: _____
_____

Notes:_____
_____
_____
_____
_____
_____
_____
_____

Additional notes on page: # _____

~ Accident / Injury Record Book ~

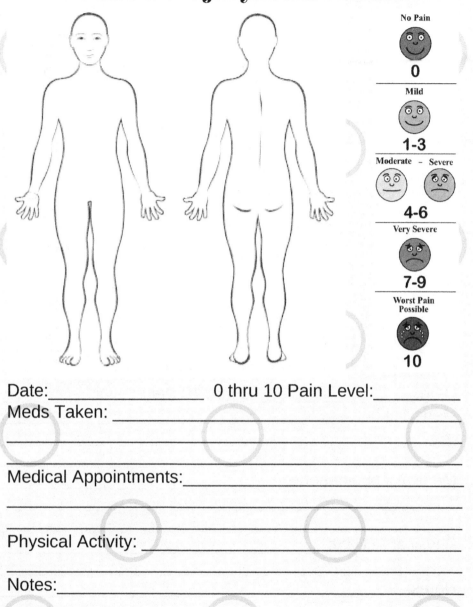

No Pain
0

Mild
1-3

Moderate – Severe
4-6

Very Severe
7-9

Worst Pain Possible
10

Date:_____ 0 thru 10 Pain Level:_____

Meds Taken: _____
_____

Medical Appointments:_____
_____

Physical Activity: _____
_____

Notes:_____
_____
_____
_____
_____
_____
_____

Additional notes on page: # _____

~ Accident / Injury Record Book ~

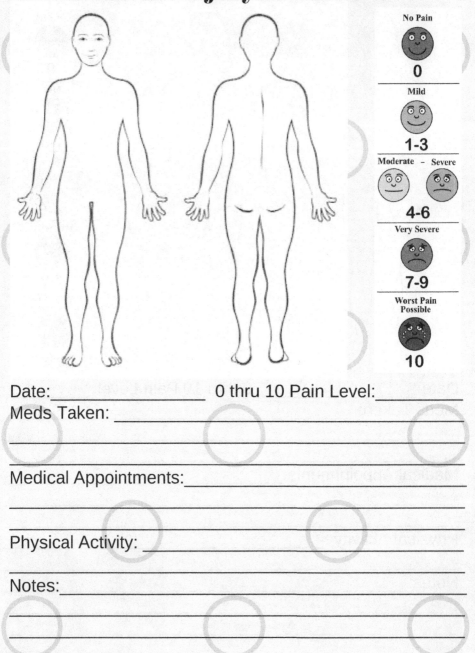

No Pain
0

Mild
1-3

Moderate – Severe
4-6

Very Severe
7-9

Worst Pain Possible
10

Date:_____ 0 thru 10 Pain Level:_____

Meds Taken: _____
_____

Medical Appointments:_____
_____
_____

Physical Activity: _____
_____

Notes:_____
_____
_____
_____
_____
_____
_____

Additional notes on page: # _____

~ Accident / Injury Record Book ~

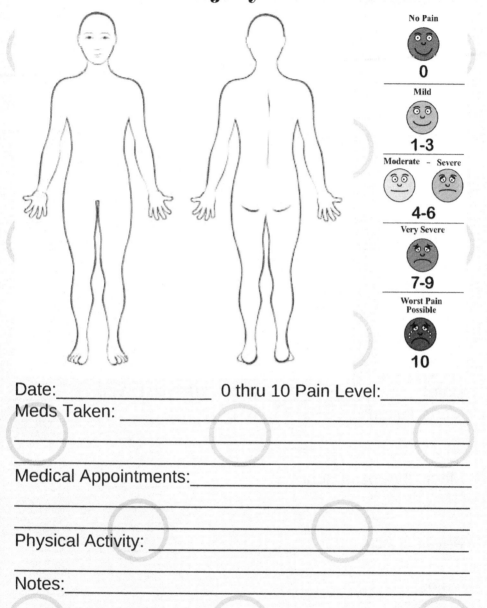

No Pain
0

Mild
1-3

Moderate – Severe
4-6

Very Severe
7-9

Worst Pain Possible
10

Date:_____ 0 thru 10 Pain Level:_____

Meds Taken: _____

_____

_____

Medical Appointments:_____

_____

_____

Physical Activity: _____

_____

Notes:_____

_____

_____

_____

_____

_____

_____

Additional notes on page: # _____

~ Accident / Injury Record Book ~

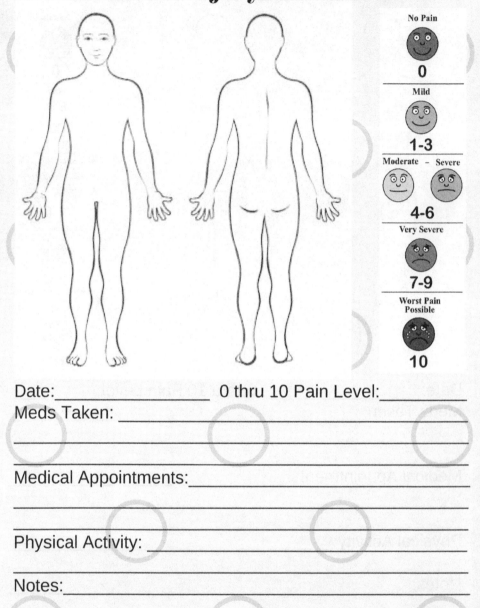

Date:_____ 0 thru 10 Pain Level:_____

Meds Taken: _____
_____

Medical Appointments:_____
_____

Physical Activity: _____
_____

Notes:_____
_____
_____
_____
_____
_____
_____

Additional notes on page: # _____

~ Accident / Injury Record Book ~

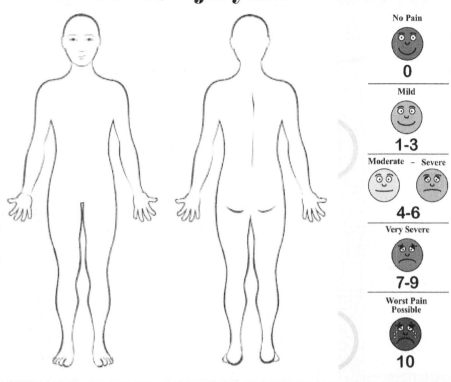

No Pain

0

Mild

1-3

Moderate – Severe

4-6

Very Severe

7-9

Worst Pain Possible

10

Date:_____ 0 thru 10 Pain Level:_____

Meds Taken: _____
_____

Medical Appointments:_____
_____

Physical Activity: _____
_____

Notes:_____
_____
_____
_____
_____
_____
_____

Additional notes on page: # _____

~ Accident / Injury Record Book ~

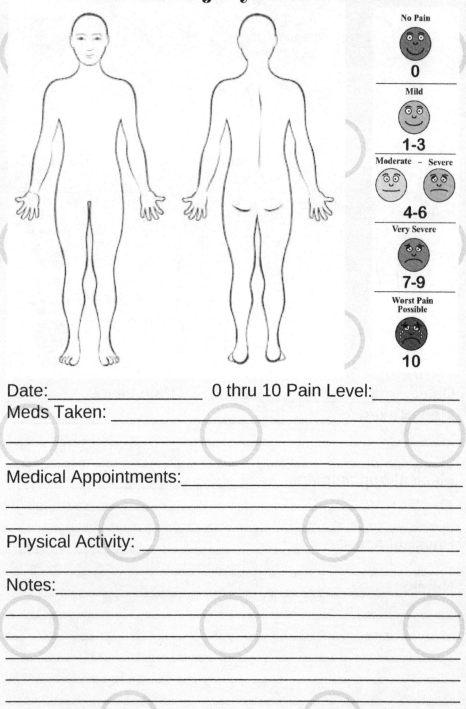

No Pain
0

Mild
1-3

Moderate – Severe
4-6

Very Severe
7-9

Worst Pain Possible
10

Date:_____ 0 thru 10 Pain Level:_____

Meds Taken: _____

_____

Medical Appointments:_____

_____

Physical Activity: _____

Notes:_____

_____

_____

_____

_____

_____

Additional notes on page: # _____

~ Accident / Injury Record Book ~

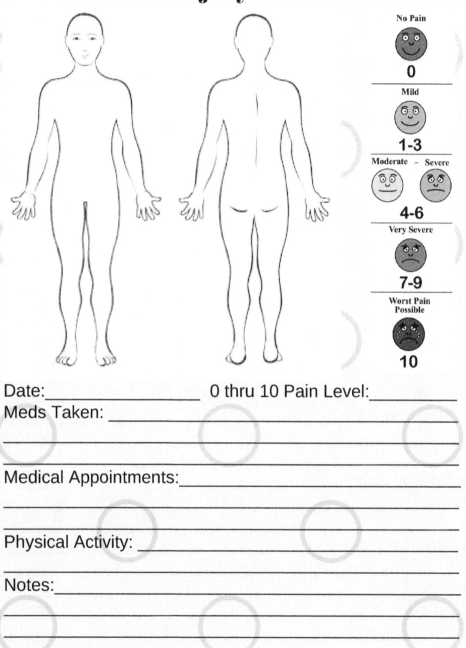

No Pain
0

Mild
1-3

Moderate – Severe
4-6

Very Severe
7-9

Worst Pain Possible
10

Date:_____ 0 thru 10 Pain Level:_____

Meds Taken: _____
_____
_____

Medical Appointments:_____
_____
_____

Physical Activity: _____
_____

Notes:_____
_____
_____
_____
_____
_____
_____
_____

Additional notes on page: # _____

~ Accident / Injury Record Book ~

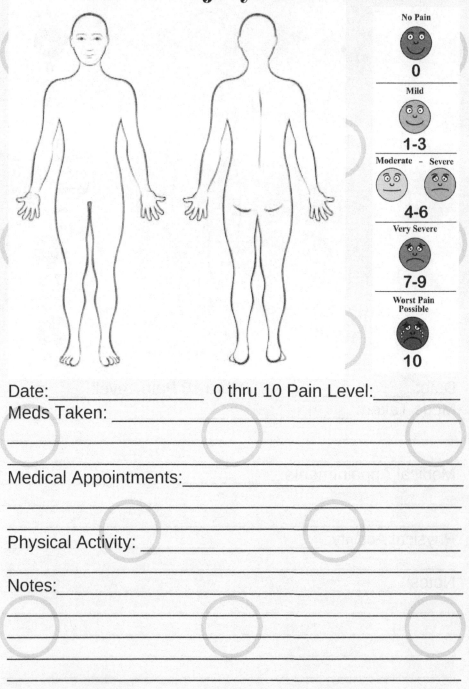

No Pain

0

Mild

1-3

Moderate – Severe

4-6

Very Severe

7-9

Worst Pain Possible

10

Date:_____ 0 thru 10 Pain Level:_____

Meds Taken: _____

_____

Medical Appointments:_____

_____

Physical Activity: _____

_____

Notes:_____

_____

_____

_____

_____

_____

_____

Additional notes on page: # _____

~ Accident / Injury Record Book ~

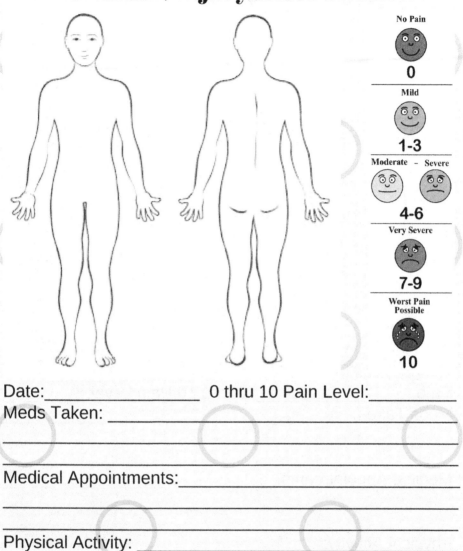

No Pain
0

Mild
1-3

Moderate – Severe
4-6

Very Severe
7-9

Worst Pain Possible
10

Date:_____ 0 thru 10 Pain Level:_____

Meds Taken: _____
_____
_____

Medical Appointments:_____
_____
_____

Physical Activity: _____
_____

Notes:_____
_____
_____
_____
_____
_____
_____

Additional notes on page: # _____

~ Accident / Injury Record Book ~

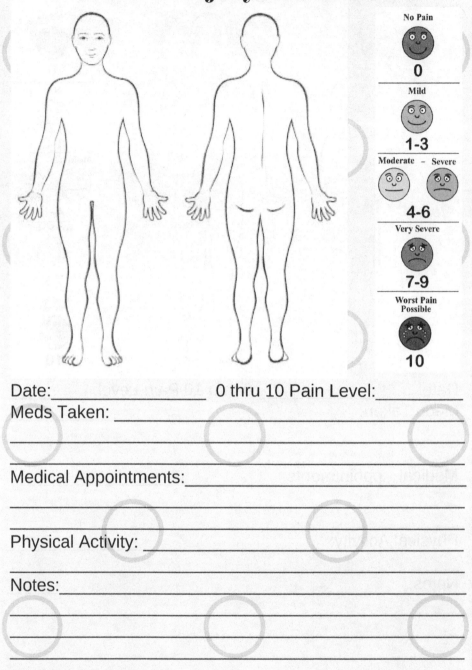

No Pain
0

Mild
1-3

Moderate – Severe
4-6

Very Severe
7-9

Worst Pain Possible
10

Date:_____ 0 thru 10 Pain Level:_____

Meds Taken: _____
_____

Medical Appointments:_____
_____
_____

Physical Activity: _____
_____

Notes:_____
_____
_____
_____
_____
_____
_____

Additional notes on page: # _____

~ Accident / Injury Record Book ~

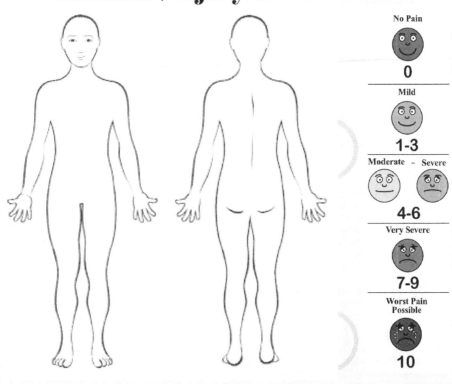

No Pain
0

Mild
1-3

Moderate – Severe
4-6

Very Severe
7-9

Worst Pain Possible
10

Date:_____ 0 thru 10 Pain Level:_____

Meds Taken: _____
_____

Medical Appointments:_____
_____

Physical Activity: _____
_____

Notes:_____
_____
_____
_____
_____
_____
_____

Additional notes on page: # _____

~ Accident / Injury Record Book ~

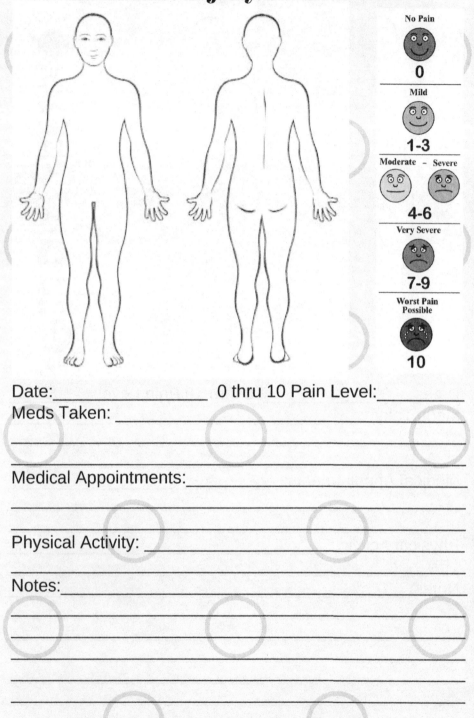

No Pain

0

Mild

1-3

Moderate – Severe

4-6

Very Severe

7-9

Worst Pain Possible

10

Date:_____ 0 thru 10 Pain Level:_____

Meds Taken: _____
_____

Medical Appointments:_____
_____

Physical Activity: _____
_____

Notes:_____
_____
_____
_____
_____
_____

Additional notes on page: # _____

~ Accident / Injury Record Book ~

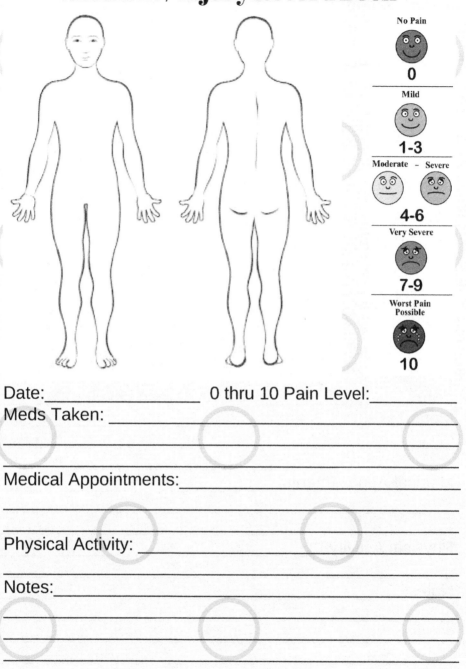

No Pain
0

Mild
1-3

Moderate – Severe
4-6

Very Severe
7-9

Worst Pain Possible
10

Date:_____ 0 thru 10 Pain Level:_____

Meds Taken: _____
_____
_____

Medical Appointments:_____
_____
_____

Physical Activity: _____
_____

Notes:_____
_____
_____
_____
_____
_____
_____

Additional notes on page: # _____

~ Accident / Injury Record Book ~

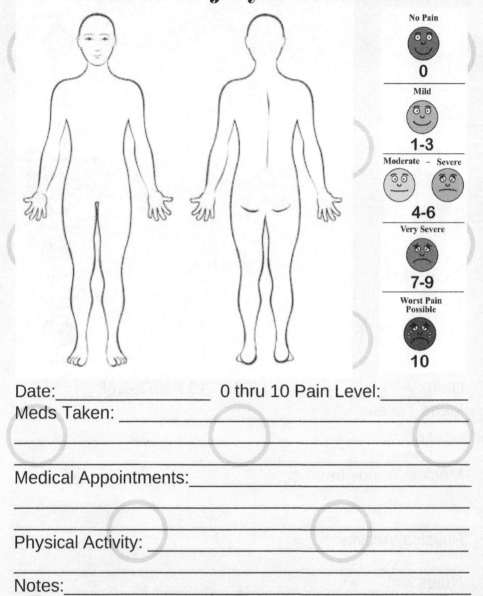

No Pain
0

Mild
1-3

Moderate – Severe
4-6

Very Severe
7-9

Worst Pain Possible
10

Date:_____ 0 thru 10 Pain Level:_____

Meds Taken: _____
_____

Medical Appointments:_____
_____

Physical Activity: _____
_____

Notes:_____
_____
_____
_____
_____
_____
_____

Additional notes on page: # _____

~ Accident / Injury Record Book ~

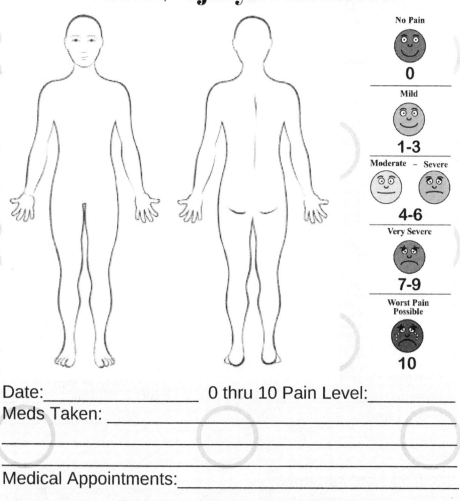

No Pain
0

Mild
1-3

Moderate – Severe
4-6

Very Severe
7-9

Worst Pain Possible
10

Date:_____ 0 thru 10 Pain Level:_____

Meds Taken: _____

_____

_____

Medical Appointments:_____

_____

_____

Physical Activity: _____

_____

Notes:_____

_____

_____

_____

_____

_____

_____

Additional notes on page: # _____

~ Accident / Injury Record Book ~

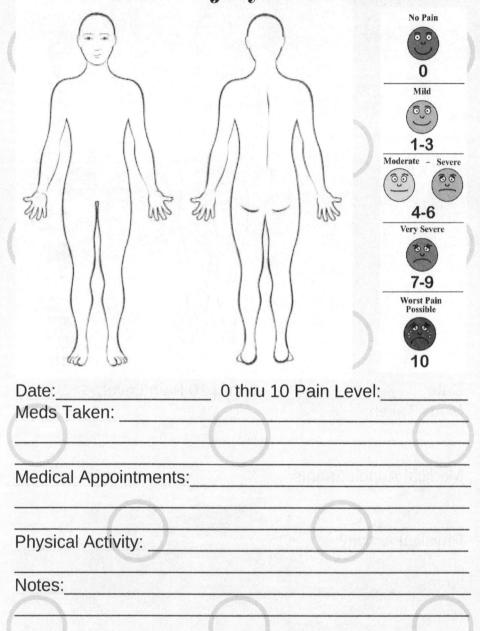

No Pain
0

Mild
1-3

Moderate - Severe
4-6

Very Severe
7-9

Worst Pain Possible
10

Date:_____ 0 thru 10 Pain Level:_____

Meds Taken: _____

_____

Medical Appointments:_____

_____

Physical Activity: _____

Notes:_____

_____

_____

_____

_____

_____

Additional notes on page: # _____

~ Accident / Injury Record Book ~

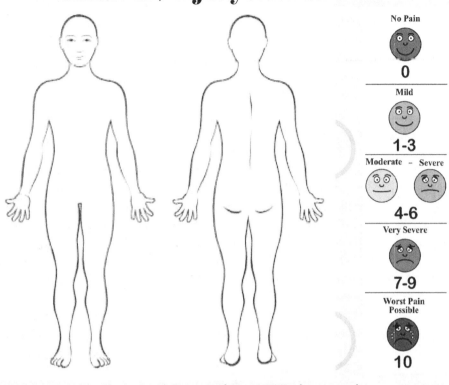

No Pain
0

Mild
1-3

Moderate – Severe
4-6

Very Severe
7-9

Worst Pain Possible
10

Date:_____ 0 thru 10 Pain Level:_____

Meds Taken: _____
_____

Medical Appointments:_____
_____

Physical Activity: _____
_____

Notes:_____
_____
_____
_____
_____
_____
_____

Additional notes on page: # _____

~ Accident / Injury Record Book ~

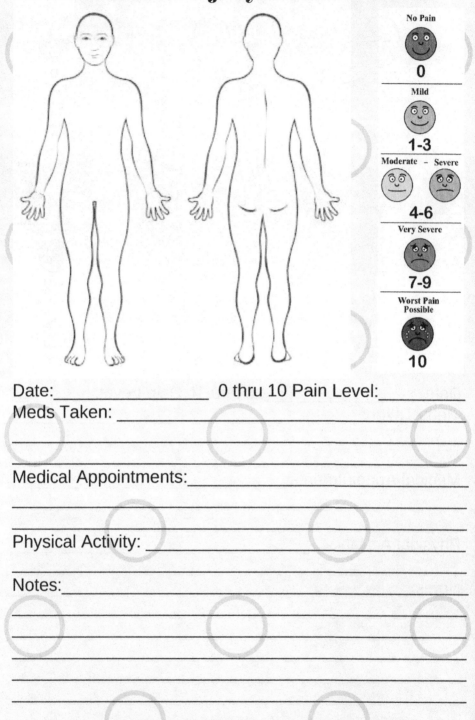

No Pain
0

Mild
1-3

Moderate – Severe
4-6

Very Severe
7-9

Worst Pain Possible
10

Date:_____ 0 thru 10 Pain Level:_____

Meds Taken: _____
_____

Medical Appointments:_____
_____

Physical Activity: _____
_____

Notes:_____
_____
_____
_____
_____
_____

Additional notes on page: # _____

~ Accident / Injury Record Book ~

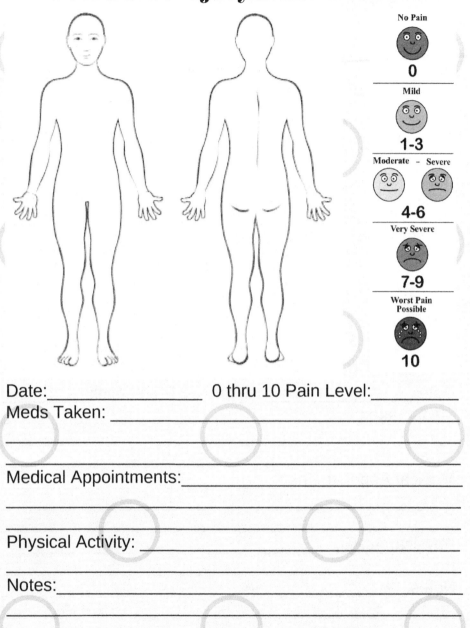

No Pain
0

Mild
1-3

Moderate – Severe
4-6

Very Severe
7-9

Worst Pain Possible
10

Date:_____ 0 thru 10 Pain Level:_____

Meds Taken: _____
_____
_____

Medical Appointments:_____
_____
_____

Physical Activity: _____
_____

Notes:_____
_____
_____
_____
_____
_____
_____

Additional notes on page: # _____

~ Accident / Injury Record Book ~

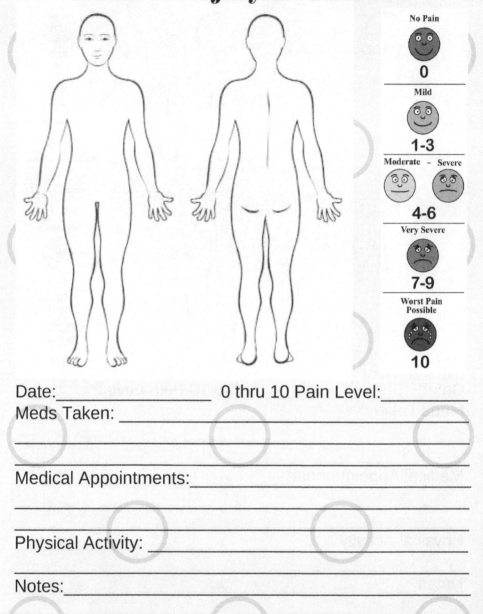

No Pain
0

Mild
1-3

Moderate – Severe
4-6

Very Severe
7-9

Worst Pain Possible
10

Date:_____ 0 thru 10 Pain Level:_____

Meds Taken: _____
_____

Medical Appointments:_____
_____

Physical Activity: _____
_____

Notes:_____
_____
_____
_____
_____
_____
_____

Additional notes on page: # _____

~ Accident / Injury Record Book ~

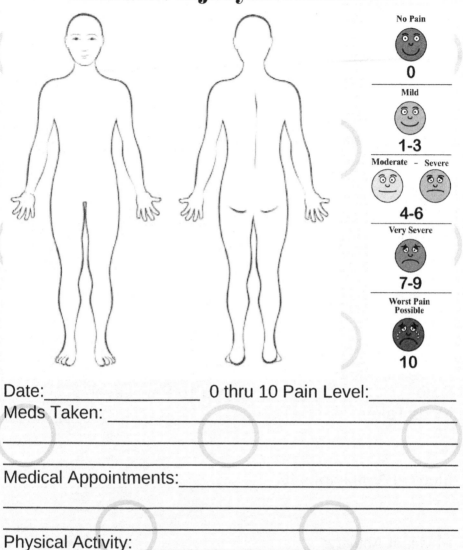

No Pain
0

Mild
1-3

Moderate – Severe
4-6

Very Severe
7-9

Worst Pain Possible
10

Date:_____ 0 thru 10 Pain Level:_____

Meds Taken: _____
_____

Medical Appointments:_____
_____

Physical Activity: _____
_____

Notes:_____
_____
_____
_____
_____
_____
_____

Additional notes on page: # _____

~ Accident / Injury Record Book ~

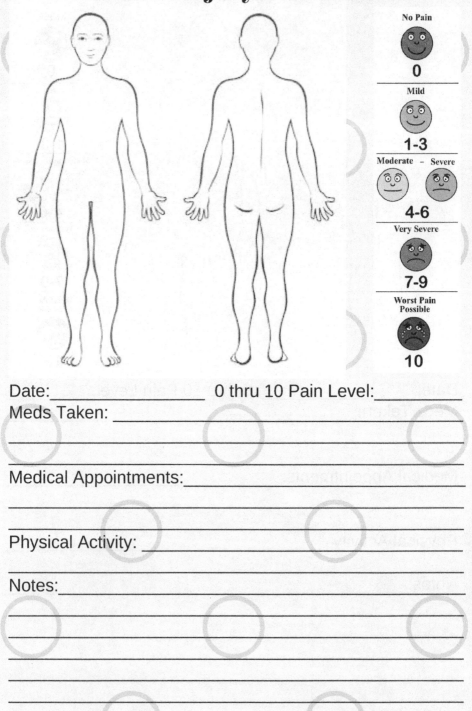

No Pain
0

Mild
1-3

Moderate – Severe
4-6

Very Severe
7-9

Worst Pain Possible
10

Date:_____ 0 thru 10 Pain Level:_____

Meds Taken: _____
_____

Medical Appointments:_____
_____
_____

Physical Activity: _____
_____

Notes:_____
_____
_____
_____
_____
_____
_____
_____

Additional notes on page: # _____

~ Accident / Injury Record Book ~

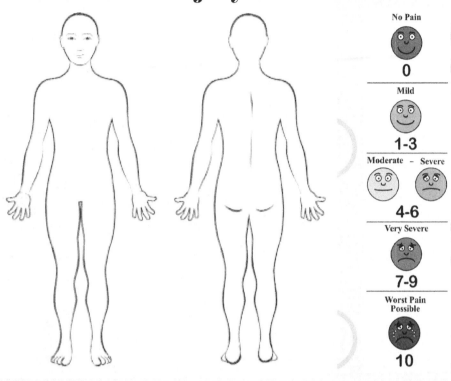

No Pain

0

Mild

1-3

Moderate – Severe

4-6

Very Severe

7-9

Worst Pain Possible

10

Date:_____ 0 thru 10 Pain Level:_____

Meds Taken: _____
_____
_____

Medical Appointments:_____
_____
_____

Physical Activity: _____
_____

Notes:_____
_____
_____
_____
_____
_____
_____
_____

Additional notes on page: # _____

~ Accident / Injury Record Book ~

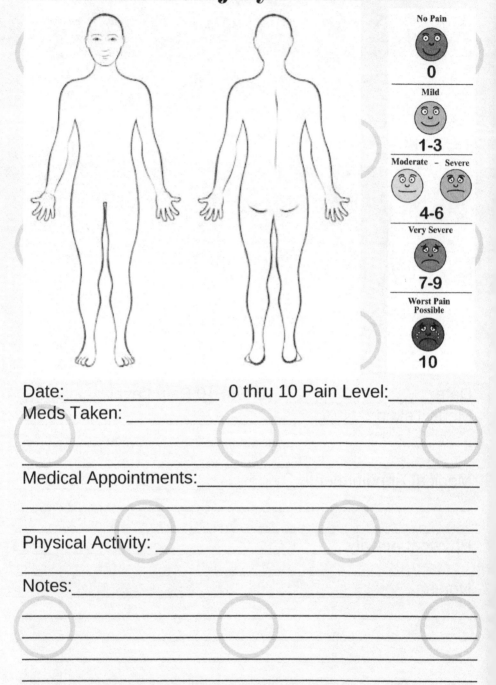

No Pain

0

Mild

1-3

Moderate – **Severe**

4-6

Very Severe

7-9

Worst Pain Possible

10

Date:_____ 0 thru 10 Pain Level:_____

Meds Taken: _____

_____

Medical Appointments:_____

_____

Physical Activity: _____

_____

Notes:_____

_____

_____

_____

_____

_____

Additional notes on page: # _____

~ Accident / Injury Record Book ~

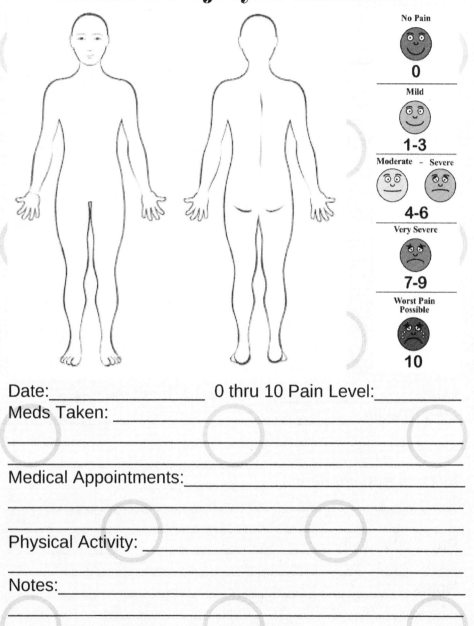

No Pain
0

Mild
1-3

Moderate – Severe
4-6

Very Severe
7-9

Worst Pain Possible
10

Date:_____ 0 thru 10 Pain Level:_____

Meds Taken: _____
_____
_____

Medical Appointments:_____
_____
_____

Physical Activity: _____
_____

Notes:_____
_____
_____
_____
_____
_____
_____

Additional notes on page: # _____

~ Accident / Injury Record Book ~

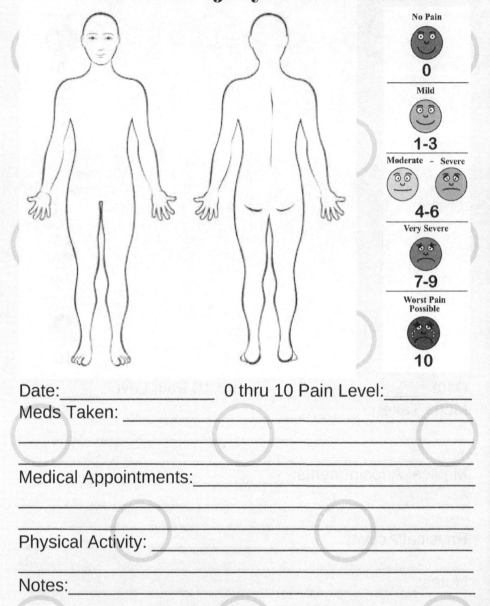

No Pain
0

Mild
1-3

Moderate – Severe
4-6

Very Severe
7-9

Worst Pain Possible
10

Date:_____ 0 thru 10 Pain Level:_____

Meds Taken: _____
_____

Medical Appointments:_____
_____

Physical Activity: _____
_____

Notes:_____
_____
_____
_____
_____
_____
_____

Additional notes on page: # _____

~ Accident / Injury Record Book ~

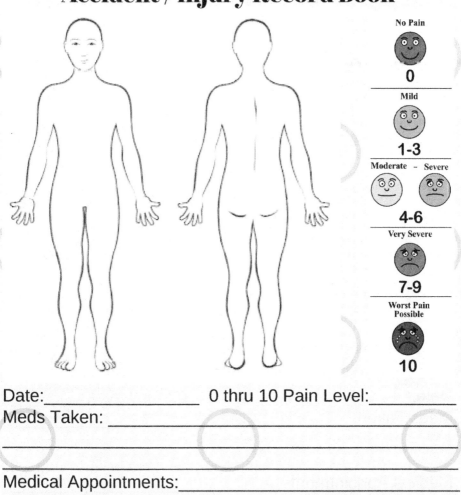

No Pain

0

Mild

1-3

Moderate – Severe

4-6

Very Severe

7-9

Worst Pain Possible

10

Date:_____ 0 thru 10 Pain Level:_____

Meds Taken: _____
_____
_____

Medical Appointments:_____
_____
_____

Physical Activity: _____
_____

Notes:_____
_____
_____
_____
_____
_____
_____

Additional notes on page: # _____

~ Accident / Injury Record Book ~

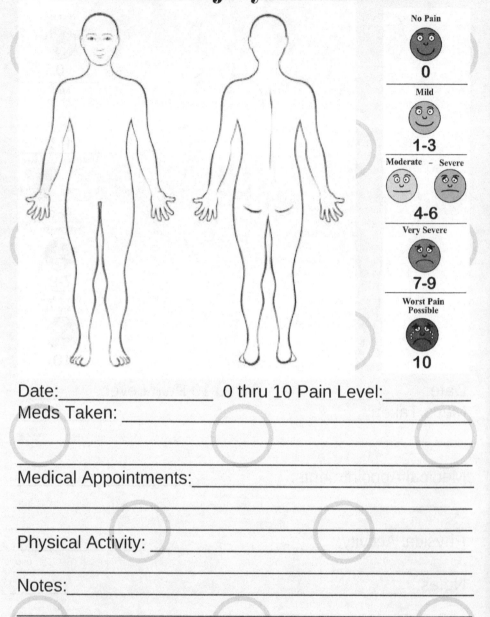

No Pain
0

Mild
1-3

Moderate – Severe
4-6

Very Severe
7-9

Worst Pain Possible
10

Date:_____ 0 thru 10 Pain Level:_____

Meds Taken: _____

_____

Medical Appointments:_____

_____

Physical Activity: _____

_____

Notes:_____

_____

_____

_____

_____

_____

_____

Additional notes on page: # _____

~ Accident / Injury Record Book ~

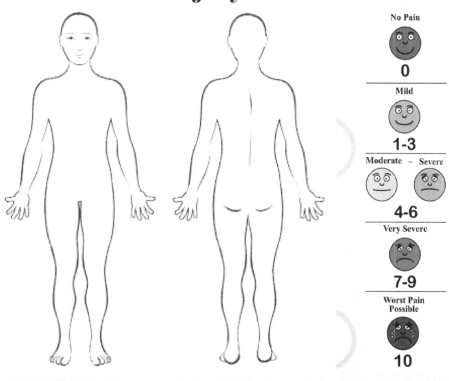

No Pain
0

Mild
1-3

Moderate – Severe
4-6

Very Severe
7-9

Worst Pain Possible
10

Date:_____ 0 thru 10 Pain Level:_____

Meds Taken: _____
_____

Medical Appointments:_____
_____

Physical Activity: _____

Notes:_____
_____
_____
_____
_____
_____
_____

Additional notes on page: # _____

~ Accident / Injury Record Book ~

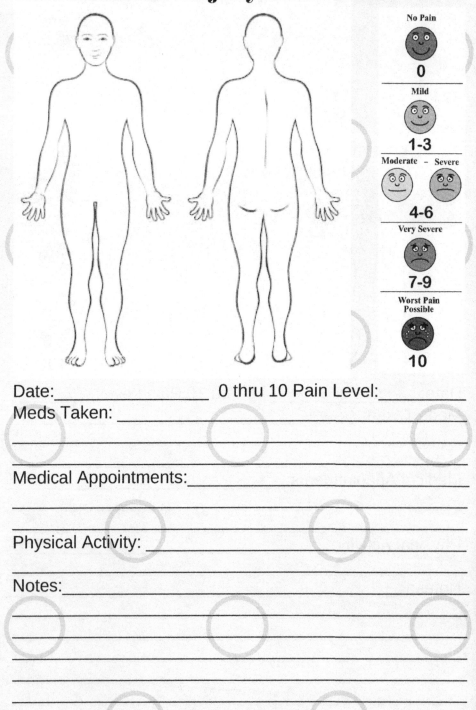

No Pain
0

Mild
1-3

Moderate – Severe
4-6

Very Severe
7-9

Worst Pain Possible
10

Date:_____ 0 thru 10 Pain Level:_____

Meds Taken: _____
_____

Medical Appointments:_____
_____
_____

Physical Activity: _____
_____

Notes:_____
_____
_____
_____
_____
_____
_____

Additional notes on page: # _____

~ Accident / Injury Record Book ~

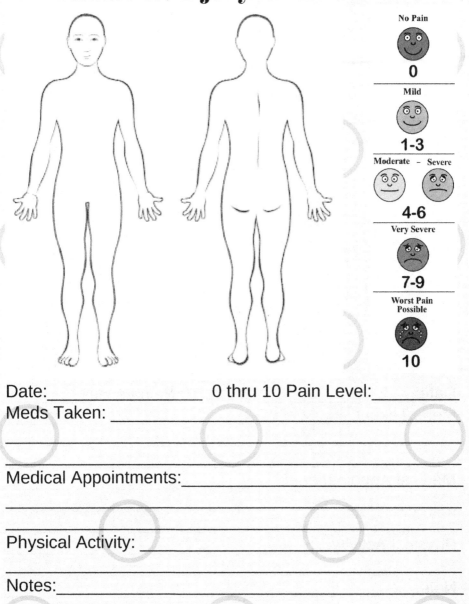

No Pain
0

Mild
1-3

Moderate – Severe
4-6

Very Severe
7-9

Worst Pain Possible
10

Date:_____ 0 thru 10 Pain Level:_____

Meds Taken: _____
_____

Medical Appointments:_____
_____

Physical Activity: _____
_____

Notes:_____
_____
_____
_____
_____
_____
_____

Additional notes on page: # _____

~ Accident / Injury Record Book ~

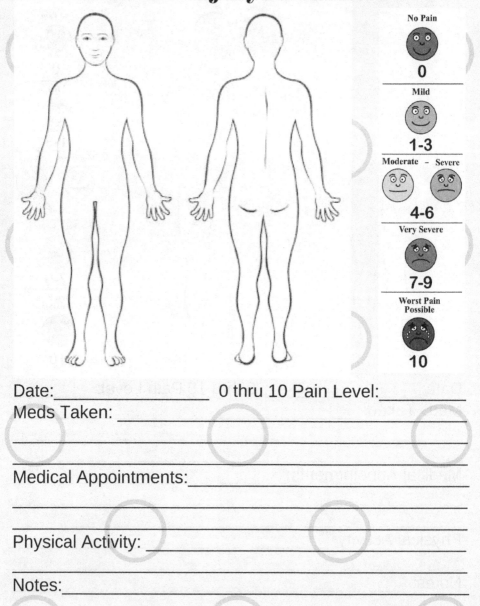

No Pain
0

Mild
1-3

Moderate – Severe
4-6

Very Severe
7-9

Worst Pain Possible
10

Date:_____ 0 thru 10 Pain Level:_____

Meds Taken: _____
_____

Medical Appointments:_____
_____

Physical Activity: _____

Notes:_____
_____
_____
_____
_____
_____
_____

Additional notes on page: # _____

~ Accident / Injury Record Book ~

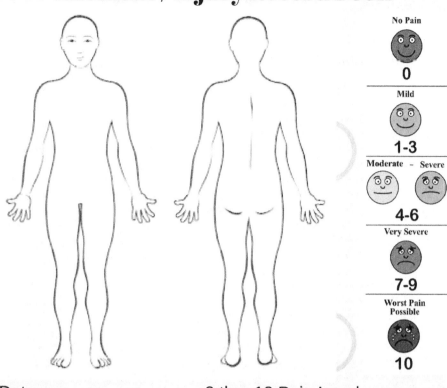

No Pain
😀 **0**

Mild
🙂 **1-3**

Moderate – Severe
😐 😟 **4-6**

Very Severe
😣 **7-9**

Worst Pain Possible
😖 **10**

Date:_____ 0 thru 10 Pain Level:_____

Meds Taken: _____

_____

Medical Appointments:_____

_____

Physical Activity: _____

Notes:_____

_____

_____

_____

_____

_____

Additional notes on page: # _____

~ Accident / Injury Record Book ~

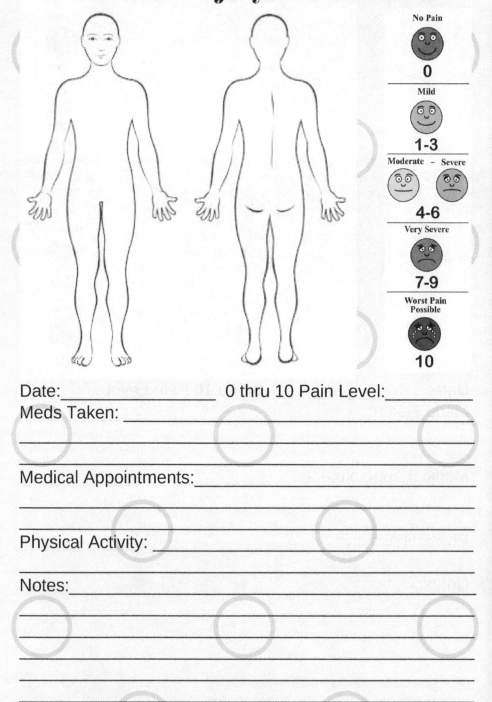

No Pain
0

Mild
1-3

Moderate – Severe
4-6

Very Severe
7-9

Worst Pain Possible
10

Date:_____ 0 thru 10 Pain Level:_____

Meds Taken: _____
_____

Medical Appointments:_____
_____

Physical Activity: _____
_____

Notes:_____
_____
_____
_____
_____
_____

Additional notes on page: # _____

~ Accident / Injury Record Book ~

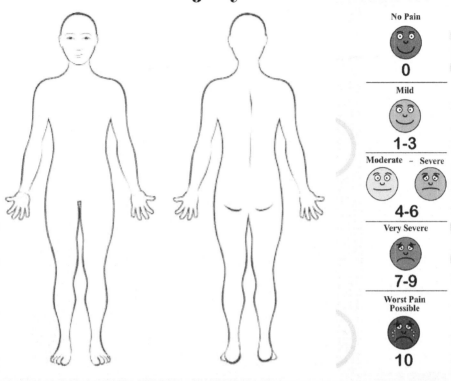

No Pain

0

Mild

1-3

Moderate – Severe

4-6

Very Severe

7-9

Worst Pain
Possible

10

Date:_____ 0 thru 10 Pain Level:_____

Meds Taken: _____
_____

Medical Appointments:_____
_____
_____

Physical Activity: _____
_____

Notes:_____
_____
_____
_____
_____
_____
_____
_____

Additional notes on page: # _____

~ Accident / Injury Record Book ~

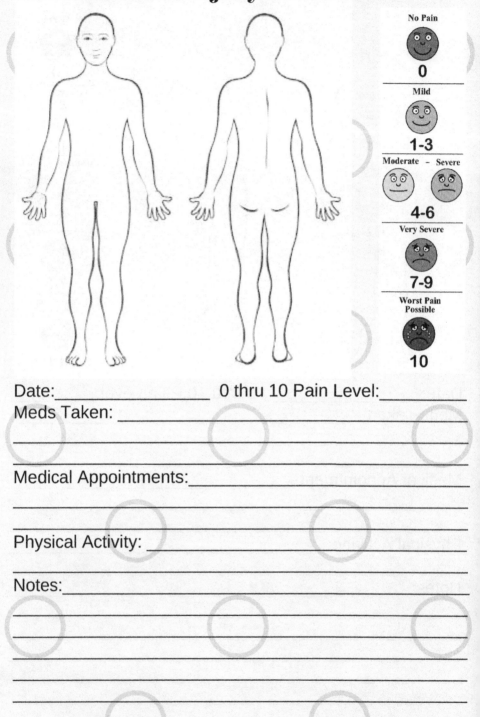

No Pain
0

Mild
1-3

Moderate – Severe
4-6

Very Severe
7-9

Worst Pain Possible
10

Date:_____ 0 thru 10 Pain Level:_____

Meds Taken: _____

_____

Medical Appointments:_____

_____

_____

Physical Activity: _____

_____

Notes:_____

_____

_____

_____

_____

_____

Additional notes on page: # _____

~ Accident / Injury Record Book ~

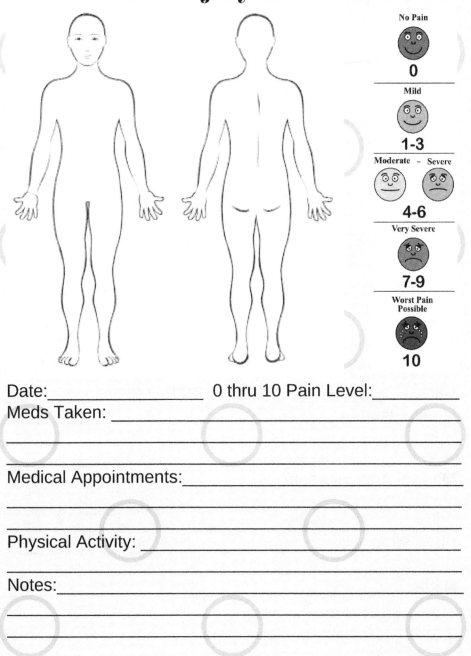

No Pain

0

Mild

1-3

Moderate – Severe

4-6

Very Severe

7-9

Worst Pain Possible

10

Date:_____ 0 thru 10 Pain Level:_____

Meds Taken: _____
_____
_____

Medical Appointments:_____
_____
_____

Physical Activity: _____
_____

Notes:_____
_____
_____
_____
_____
_____
_____
_____

Additional notes on page: # _____

~ Accident / Injury Record Book ~

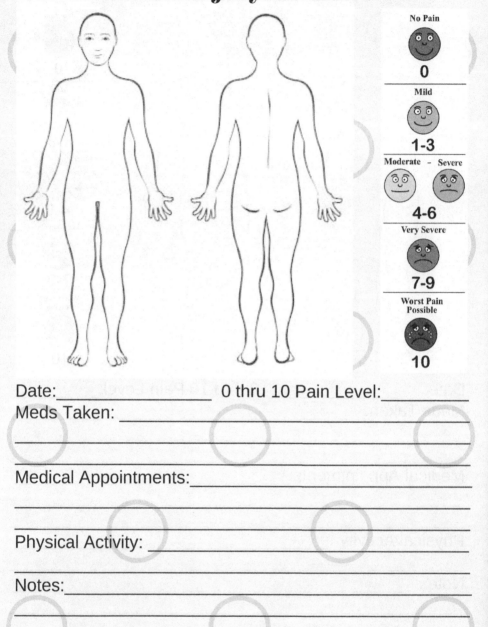

No Pain
0

Mild
1-3

Moderate – Severe
4-6

Very Severe
7-9

Worst Pain Possible
10

Date:_____ 0 thru 10 Pain Level:_____

Meds Taken: _____
_____

Medical Appointments:_____
_____
_____

Physical Activity: _____
_____

Notes:_____
_____
_____
_____
_____
_____
_____

Additional notes on page: # _____

~ Accident / Injury Record Book ~

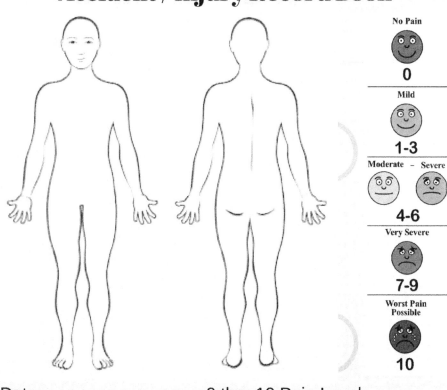

No Pain
0

Mild
1-3

Moderate – Severe
4-6

Very Severe
7-9

Worst Pain Possible
10

Date:_____ 0 thru 10 Pain Level:_____

Meds Taken: _____
_____

Medical Appointments:_____
_____

Physical Activity: _____
_____

Notes:_____
_____
_____
_____
_____
_____
_____

Additional notes on page: # _____

~ Accident / Injury Record Book ~

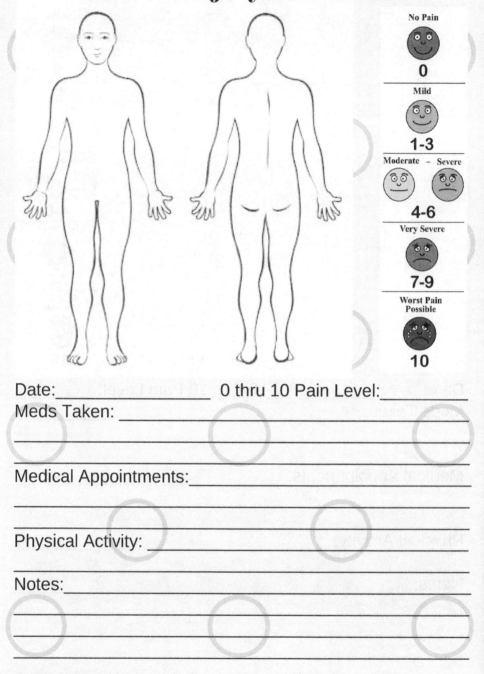

No Pain
0

Mild
1-3

Moderate – Severe
4-6

Very Severe
7-9

Worst Pain Possible
10

Date:_____ 0 thru 10 Pain Level:_____

Meds Taken: _____
_____

Medical Appointments:_____
_____
_____

Physical Activity: _____
_____

Notes:_____
_____
_____
_____
_____
_____
_____

Additional notes on page: # _____

~ Accident / Injury Record Book ~

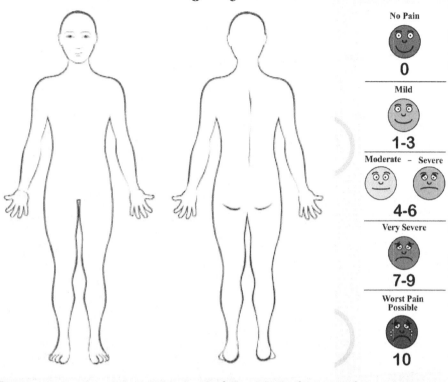

No Pain
0

Mild
1-3

Moderate – Severe
4-6

Very Severe
7-9

Worst Pain Possible
10

Date:_____ 0 thru 10 Pain Level:_____

Meds Taken: _____

_____

_____

Medical Appointments:_____

_____

_____

Physical Activity: _____

_____

Notes:_____

_____

_____

_____

_____

_____

_____

_____

Additional notes on page: # _____

~ Accident / Injury Record Book ~

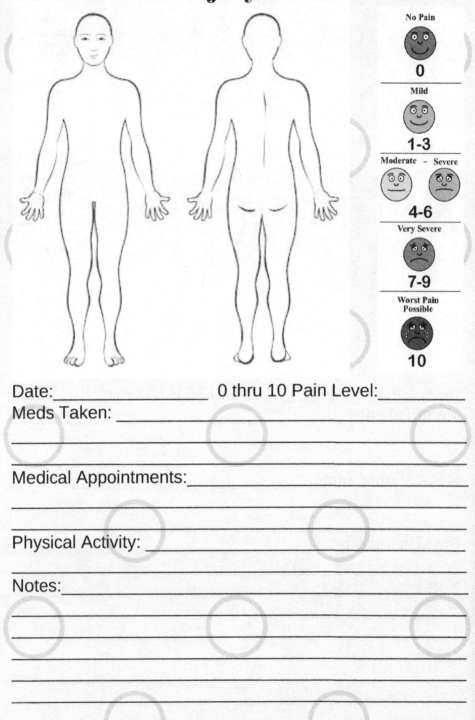

No Pain
0

Mild
1-3

Moderate – Severe
4-6

Very Severe
7-9

Worst Pain Possible
10

Date:_____ 0 thru 10 Pain Level:_____

Meds Taken: _____

_____

Medical Appointments:_____

_____

Physical Activity: _____

_____

Notes:_____

_____

_____

_____

_____

_____

_____

Additional notes on page: # _____

~ Accident / Injury Record Book ~

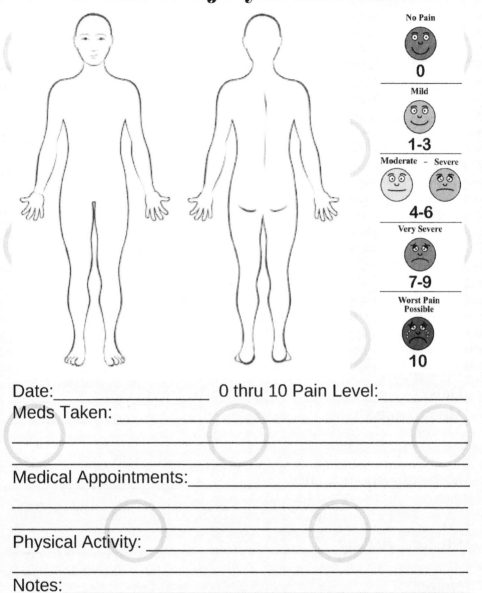

No Pain
0

Mild
1-3

Moderate – Severe
4-6

Very Severe
7-9

Worst Pain Possible
10

Date:_____ 0 thru 10 Pain Level:_____

Meds Taken: _____
_____

Medical Appointments:_____
_____

Physical Activity: _____
_____

Notes:_____
_____
_____
_____
_____
_____
_____

Additional notes on page: # _____

~ Accident / Injury Record Book ~

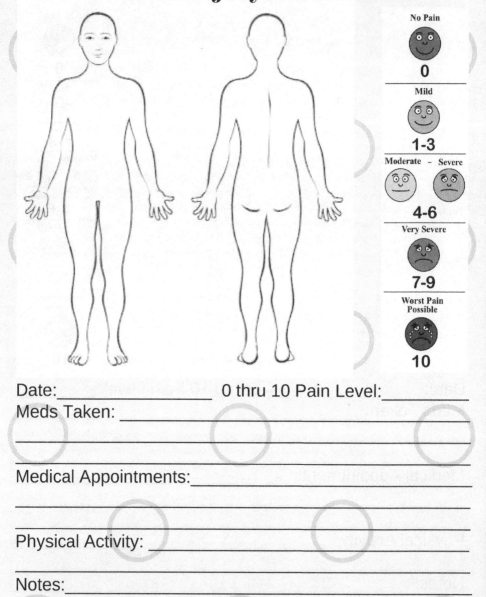

No Pain
0

Mild
1-3

Moderate – Severe
4-6

Very Severe
7-9

Worst Pain Possible
10

Date:_____ 0 thru 10 Pain Level:_____

Meds Taken: _____
_____

Medical Appointments:_____
_____

Physical Activity: _____
_____

Notes:_____
_____
_____
_____
_____
_____
_____

Additional notes on page: # _____

~ Accident / Injury Record Book ~

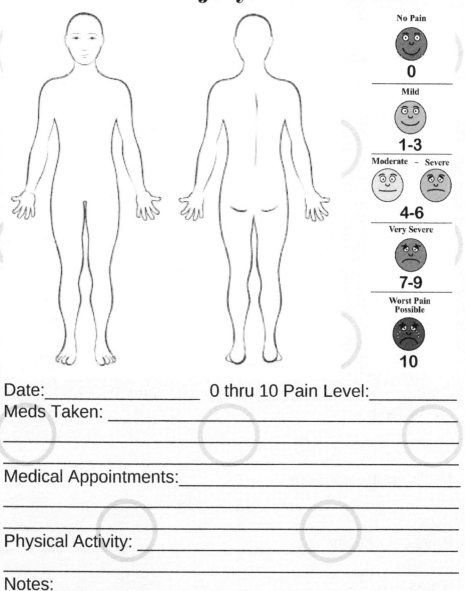

No Pain

0

Mild

1-3

Moderate – Severe

4-6

Very Severe

7-9

Worst Pain Possible

10

Date:_____ 0 thru 10 Pain Level:_____

Meds Taken: _____

_____

_____

Medical Appointments:_____

_____

Physical Activity: _____

_____

Notes:_____

_____

_____

_____

_____

_____

_____

Additional notes on page: # _____

~ Accident / Injury Record Book ~

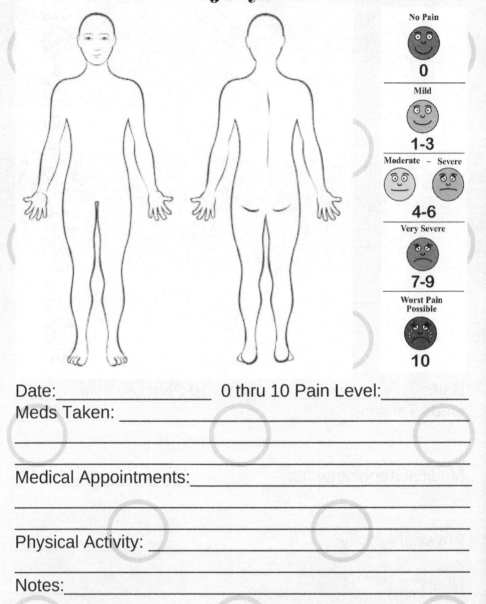

No Pain
0

Mild
1-3

Moderate – Severe
4-6

Very Severe
7-9

Worst Pain Possible
10

Date:_____ 0 thru 10 Pain Level:_____

Meds Taken: _____
_____

Medical Appointments:_____
_____

Physical Activity: _____
_____

Notes:_____
_____
_____
_____
_____
_____
_____

Additional notes on page: # _____

~ Accident / Injury Record Book ~

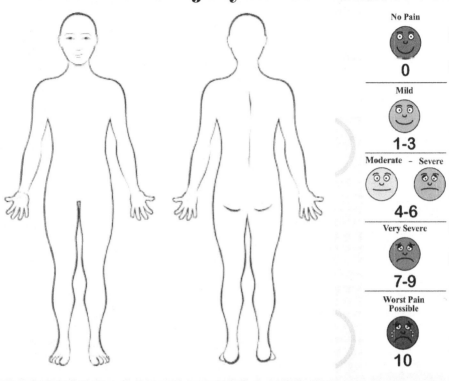

No Pain
0

Mild
1-3

Moderate - Severe
4-6

Very Severe
7-9

Worst Pain Possible
10

Date:_____ 0 thru 10 Pain Level:_____

Meds Taken: _____
_____
_____

Medical Appointments:_____
_____
_____

Physical Activity: _____
_____

Notes:_____
_____
_____
_____
_____
_____
_____

Additional notes on page: # _____

~ Accident / Injury Record Book ~

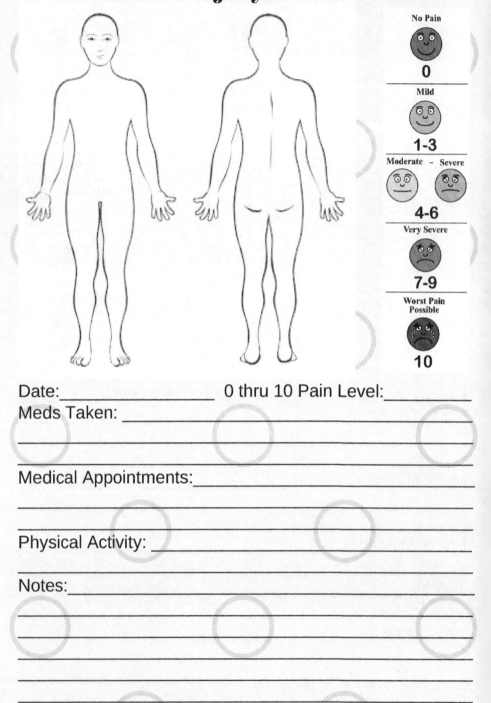

No Pain
0

Mild
1-3

Moderate – Severe
4-6

Very Severe
7-9

Worst Pain Possible
10

Date:_____ 0 thru 10 Pain Level:_____

Meds Taken: _____
_____

Medical Appointments:_____
_____

Physical Activity: _____

Notes:_____
_____
_____
_____
_____
_____

Additional notes on page: # _____

~ Accident / Injury Record Book ~

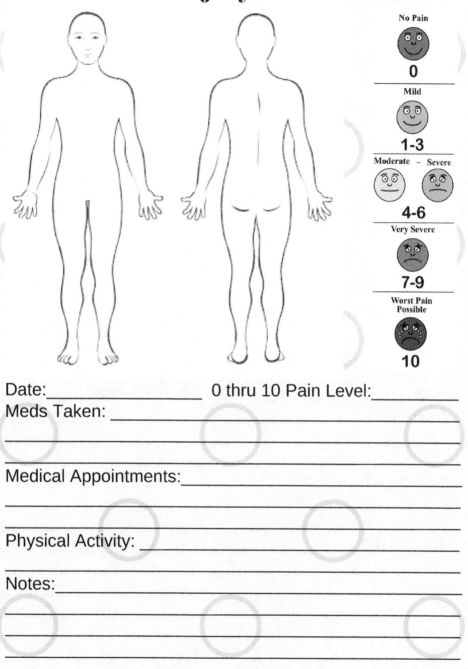

No Pain
0

Mild
1-3

Moderate – Severe
4-6

Very Severe
7-9

Worst Pain Possible
10

Date:_____ 0 thru 10 Pain Level:_____

Meds Taken: _____
_____
_____

Medical Appointments:_____
_____
_____

Physical Activity: _____
_____

Notes:_____
_____
_____
_____
_____
_____
_____

Additional notes on page: # _____

~ Accident / Injury Record Book ~

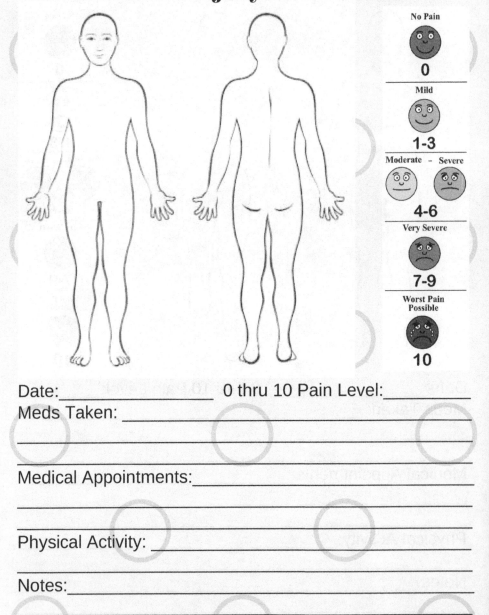

No Pain
0

Mild
1-3

Moderate - Severe
4-6

Very Severe
7-9

Worst Pain Possible
10

Date:_____ 0 thru 10 Pain Level:_____

Meds Taken: _____
_____

Medical Appointments:_____
_____
_____

Physical Activity: _____
_____

Notes:_____
_____
_____
_____
_____
_____
_____

Additional notes on page: # _____

~ Accident / Injury Record Book ~

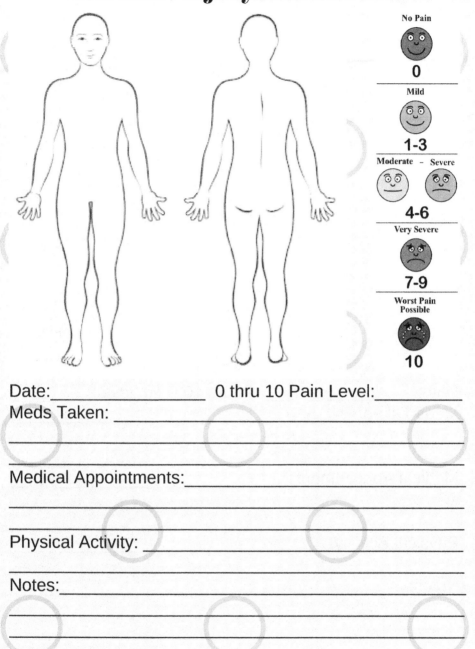

No Pain
0

Mild
1-3

Moderate – Severe
4-6

Very Severe
7-9

Worst Pain Possible
10

Date:_____ 0 thru 10 Pain Level:_____

Meds Taken: _____
_____
_____

Medical Appointments:_____
_____
_____

Physical Activity: _____
_____

Notes:_____
_____
_____
_____
_____
_____
_____

Additional notes on page: # _____

~ Accident / Injury Record Book ~

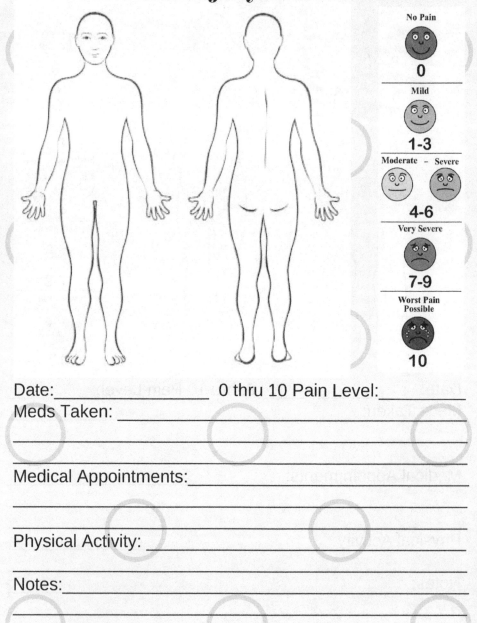

Date:_____ 0 thru 10 Pain Level:_____

Meds Taken: _____

_____

Medical Appointments:_____

_____

Physical Activity: _____

_____

Notes:_____

_____

_____

_____

_____

_____

_____

Additional notes on page: # _____

~ Accident / Injury Record Book ~

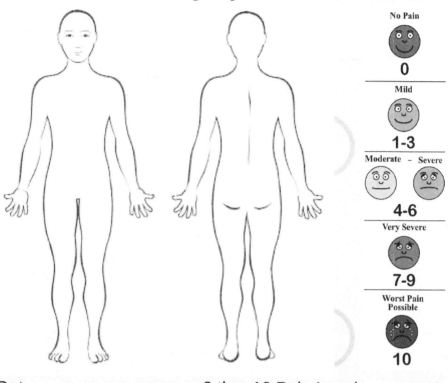

No Pain
0

Mild
1-3

Moderate – Severe
4-6

Very Severe
7-9

Worst Pain Possible
10

Date:_____ 0 thru 10 Pain Level:_____

Meds Taken: _____
_____

Medical Appointments:_____
_____
_____

Physical Activity: _____
_____

Notes:_____
_____
_____
_____
_____
_____
_____

Additional notes on page: # _____

~ Accident / Injury Record Book ~

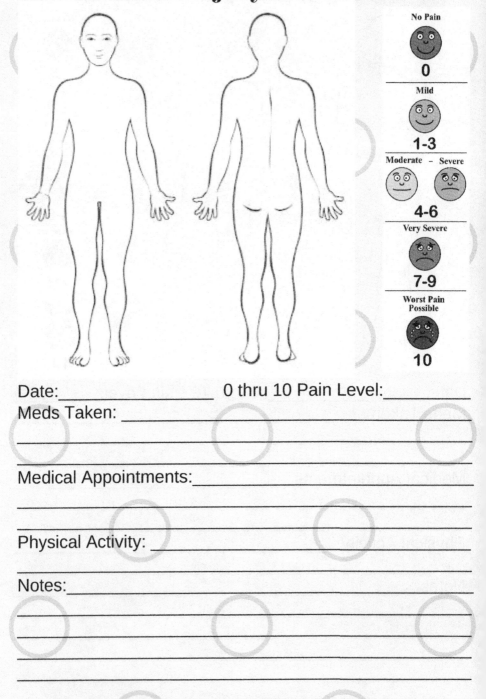

No Pain
0

Mild
1-3

Moderate – Severe
4-6

Very Severe
7-9

Worst Pain Possible
10

Date:_____ 0 thru 10 Pain Level:_____

Meds Taken: _____
_____

Medical Appointments:_____
_____

Physical Activity: _____
_____

Notes:_____
_____
_____
_____
_____
_____
_____

Additional notes on page: # _____

~ Accident / Injury Record Book ~

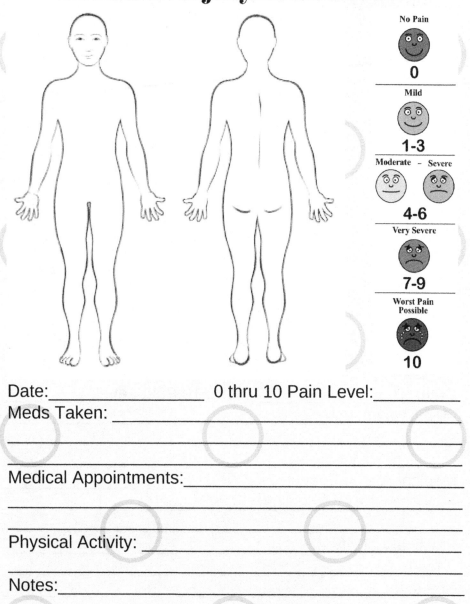

No Pain
0

Mild
1-3

Moderate – Severe
4-6

Very Severe
7-9

Worst Pain Possible
10

Date:_____ 0 thru 10 Pain Level:_____

Meds Taken: _____
_____
_____

Medical Appointments:_____
_____
_____

Physical Activity: _____
_____

Notes:_____
_____
_____
_____
_____
_____
_____

Additional notes on page: # _____

~ Accident / Injury Record Book ~

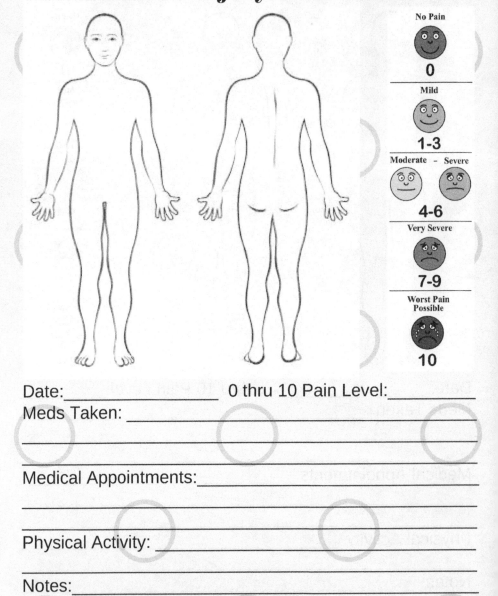

No Pain	0
Mild	1-3
Moderate – Severe	4-6
Very Severe	7-9
Worst Pain Possible	10

Date:_____ 0 thru 10 Pain Level:_____

Meds Taken: _____
_____

Medical Appointments:_____
_____
_____

Physical Activity: _____
_____

Notes:_____
_____
_____
_____
_____
_____
_____

Additional notes on page: # _____

~ Accident / Injury Record Book ~

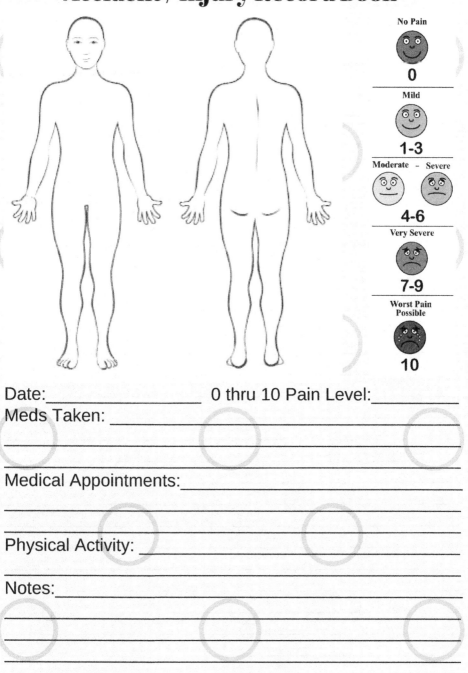

No Pain
0

Mild
1-3

Moderate – Severe
4-6

Very Severe
7-9

Worst Pain Possible
10

Date:_____ 0 thru 10 Pain Level:_____

Meds Taken: _____
_____
_____

Medical Appointments:_____
_____
_____

Physical Activity: _____
_____

Notes:_____
_____
_____
_____
_____
_____
_____
_____

Additional notes on page: # _____

~ Accident / Injury Record Book ~

Additional Notes: _____

_____

_____

_____

_____

_____

_____

_____

_____

_____

_____

_____

_____

_____

_____

_____

_____

_____

_____

_____

_____

_____

_____

_____

_____

_____

_____

_____

~ Accident / Injury Record Book ~

Additional Notes: _____

_____

_____

_____

_____

_____

_____

_____

_____

_____

_____

_____

_____

_____

_____

_____

_____

_____

_____

_____

_____

_____

~ Accident / Injury Record Book ~

Additional Notes: _____

_____

_____

_____

_____

_____

_____

_____

_____

_____

_____

_____

_____

_____

_____

_____

_____

_____

_____

_____

_____

_____

_____

~ Accident / Injury Record Book ~

Additional Notes: _____

~ Accident / Injury Record Book ~

Additional Notes: _____

_____

_____

_____

_____

_____

_____

_____

_____

_____

_____

_____

_____

_____

_____

_____

_____

_____

_____

_____

_____

_____

_____

_____

~ Accident / Injury Record Book ~

Additional Notes: _____

~ Accident / Injury Record Book ~

Additional Notes: _____

~ Accident / Injury Record Book ~

Additional Notes: _____

_____

_____

_____

_____

_____

_____

_____

_____

_____

_____

_____

_____

_____

_____

_____

_____

_____

_____

_____

_____

_____

_____

_____

~ Accident / Injury Record Book ~

Additional Notes: _____

~ Accident / Injury Record Book ~

Additional Notes: _____

_____

_____

_____

_____

_____

_____

_____

_____

_____

_____

_____

_____

_____

_____

_____

_____

_____

_____

_____

_____

_____

_____

_____

_____

_____

_____

_____

~ Accident / Injury Record Book ~

Additional Notes: _____

_____

_____

_____

_____

_____

_____

_____

_____

_____

_____

_____

_____

_____

_____

_____

_____

_____

_____

_____

_____

_____

_____

_____

_____

_____

~ Accident / Injury Record Book ~

Additional Notes: _____

_____

_____

_____

_____

_____

_____

_____

_____

_____

_____

_____

_____

_____

_____

_____

_____

_____

_____

_____

_____

_____

_____

_____

_____

_____

_____

_____

_____

~ Accident / Injury Record Book ~

Additional Notes: _____

~ Accident / Injury Record Book ~

Additional Notes: _____

_____

_____

_____

_____

_____

_____

_____

_____

_____

_____

_____

_____

_____

_____

_____

_____

_____

_____

_____

_____

_____

_____

_____

_____

_____

~ Accident / Injury Record Book ~

Additional Notes: _____

~ Accident / Injury Record Book ~

Additional Notes: _____

_____

_____

_____

_____

_____

_____

_____

_____

_____

_____

_____

_____

_____

_____

_____

_____

_____

_____

_____

_____

_____

_____

_____

_____

_____

_____

_____

~ Accident / Injury Record Book ~

Additional Notes: _____

_____
_____
_____
_____
_____
_____
_____
_____
_____
_____
_____
_____
_____
_____
_____
_____
_____
_____
_____
_____
_____
_____
_____
_____
_____

~ Accident / Injury Record Book ~

Additional Notes: _____

~ Accident / Injury Record Book ~

Additional Notes: _____

~ Accident / Injury Record Book ~

Additional Notes: _____

_____

_____

_____

_____

_____

_____

_____

_____

_____

_____

_____

_____

_____

_____

_____

_____

_____

_____

_____

_____

_____

_____

_____

_____

_____

_____

_____

_____

~ Accident / Injury Record Book ~

Additional Notes: _____

_____

_____

_____

_____

_____

_____

_____

_____

_____

_____

_____

_____

_____

_____

_____

_____

_____

_____

_____

_____

_____

_____

_____

_____

_____

_____

_____

_____

_____

~ Accident / Injury Record Book ~

Additional Notes: _____

_____
_____
_____
_____
_____
_____
_____
_____
_____
_____
_____
_____
_____
_____
_____
_____
_____
_____
_____
_____
_____
_____
_____
_____
_____
_____

~ Accident / Injury Record Book ~

Additional Notes: _____

_____

_____

_____

_____

_____

_____

_____

_____

_____

_____

_____

_____

_____

_____

_____

_____

_____

_____

_____

_____

_____

_____

_____

_____

_____

_____

~ Accident / Injury Record Book ~

Additional Notes: _____

_____

_____

_____

_____

_____

_____

_____

_____

_____

_____

_____

_____

_____

_____

_____

_____

_____

_____

_____

_____

_____

_____

_____

_____

_____

_____

_____

_____

_____

~ Accident / Injury Record Book ~

Additional Notes: _____

_____
_____
_____
_____
_____
_____
_____
_____
_____
_____
_____
_____
_____
_____
_____
_____
_____
_____
_____
_____
_____
_____
_____
_____
_____
_____
_____
_____
_____
_____
_____

~ Accident / Injury Record Book ~

Additional Notes: _____

~ List important websites here ~

~ List important email addresses here ~

Other books or projects written or created by Kenneth R. McClelland, that are available in ebook or paperback format, through amazon.com and elsewhere.

~ For the Little People ~

The Jade Lion
Harmony Farms
Different Friends
Finding Grandma
Terry's Round House
The ABC's of African American Inventions
Another Chicken Story: The Stranger Danger

~ For the Bigger People ~

The Slave's Diary
My Lupus Journal
The Pandemic Report
The Chronic Pain Journal
My Fibromyalgia Journal
My Fibromyalgia Journal - Lite
The Chronic Pain Journal - Lite
The Pandemic Preparedness Guide
Accident / Injury Record Book * Legal
House Flipping & Home Remodel Journal
How to Make Your Water Heater Last Longer

http://teslatoys.wixsite.com/stranger-danger

Made in the USA
Las Vegas, NV
30 April 2024

89322654R00080